Advance Acclaim for The Working Womb

EYE-OPENING. I AM IN AWE READING THIS BOOK. The mix of medicine with personal experiences is unique. If I knew these facts when I got pregnant, I would have taken better care of myself and my fetus. Highly informative, compassionate ...pioneering ideas and innovative applications ... empathy for patients ... tremendous medical detail and difficult concepts presented in simple terms ... understanding becomes easy.

—Dr Litsa Kranias, PhD, Fellow of the American Heart Association; Hanna Professor, Director of Cardiovascular Biology & Distinguished University Research Professor, Department of Pharmacology & Systems Physiology, University of Cincinnati College of Medicine

REMARKABLE... For women and their partners who have experienced multiple miscarriages and ask 'why does this keep happening?' But importantly, this book is ultimately also for open-minded obstetricians who are willing to consider new pathways to help their patients. As a medical doctor, I confess that we learned next to nothing about the placenta in medical school...Dr Kofinas, having devoted his career to understanding this orphan organ, shares his experience on how to diagnose and treat the most common placental problems that lead to miscarriage. I have had the incredible privilege to be under Dr Kofinas's care for two tenuous but ultimately healthy pregnancies after six prior miscarriages. **THIS BOOK IS LIKE BEING IN HIS OFFICE...** instead of patronizing pregnant women, it refreshingly provides them with medical knowledge to understand their placentas and advocate for better care.

—Dr Umut Sarpel, MD, Fellow of the American College of Surgeons; Associate Professor of Surgery, Division of Surgical Oncology & Hepatobiliary Surgery, Icahn School of Medicine at Mount Sinai; Director, General Surgery Program, Icahn School of Medicine at Mount Sinai (Morningside/West)

I HIGHLY RECOMMEND THE WORKING WOMB, an informative book specifically for an often forgotten group: women having difficult pregnancies. Dr Kofinas explains the placenta science that underlies many pregnancy problems in language that's easy to understand. The cases he presents from his files will give readers much-needed hope, by showing them how others have endured similar problems and succeeded.

—Dr Lorraine Chrisomalis-Valasiadis, MD, obstetrician and gynecologist, New York City, Adjunct Professor of Obstetrics and Gynecology, Northwell Health (New York State's largest healthcare provider)

Dr Kofinas has done a great job in producing a book that explains, in language that will be understandable to people with no medical background, the very complex development process and vital role of the placenta, in pregnancy and in the health of both the baby and the mother. He is **A MODERN RENAISSANCE MAN.**

—Dr James C Rose, PhD, Emeritus Director, Center for Research in Obstetrics and Gynecology, Wake Forest Baptist Medical Center, Winston-Salem, North Carolina

The
WORKING
WOMB

How proven placenta science can empower you to conquer pregnancy anguish, triumph over miscarriage, and have a thriving baby!

Alexander Kofinas, MD

Associate Professor of Clinical Obstetrics & Gynecology
Weill Cornell Medicine, Cornell University, New York

MONTAGU HOUSE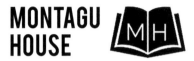

Montagu House is an imprint of Asher Associates Publishing, 16225 Dark Hollow Road, Upperco, Baltimore County, Maryland 21155, United States of America. Editorial and production offices: 254 Commercial Street, Merrill's Wharf Suite 245, Portland, Maine 04101. For all inquiries please write to editorial@montaguhouse.com

The Montagu House colophon, representing an open book bearing the initials 'MH' is a commercial mark of Asher Associates.

You must not circulate this book in any other binding or cover and you must impose the same condition on any acquirer.

This publication and all parts thereof are protected by copyright. All rights reserved. Any use of it outside the strict provisions of the copyright law without consent of the publisher is forbidden and will incur penalties. No part of this book may be reproduced or transmitted in any form or by any means, electronic or mechanical, including photocopying, recording or by any information storage and retrieval system, without written permission from the publisher, except for the inclusion of brief quotations in a review.

Copyright © Alexander Kofinas 2020. Printed in the United States of America.

LCCN: 2019954680

ISBN: 978-0-9823734-5-3

BISAC: MED033000

MEDICAL / Gynecology & Obstetrics; MED070000   MEDICAL / Perinatology & Neonatology; MED082000   MEDICAL / Reproductive Medicine & Technology; BUS033040   BUSINESS & ECONOMICS / Insurance / Health

ACKNOWLEDGEMENTS AND DEDICATION

A book of this kind necessarily reflects debts both personal and professional. In my case, these stretch across a lifetime. This book would not exist without the encouragement and support of my family, from my childhood to the present day. Additionally, I am lastingly grateful to my teachers and mentors through the years for the knowledge that made it possible for me to become a physician; to my clinical and academic colleagues for endless intellectual stimulation and lively exchanges of ideas; to my students for showing me how much teachers can learn from their pupils; to my staff, past and present, for their diligent support, often well beyond the call of duty; and to Mr N J Slabbert for sharing with me his insight into the art of science writing. Above all, I record my thanks beyond measure to my patients, who have entrusted their pregnancy problems to me, enriching my life and understanding with their courage and resolve. To them I humbly dedicate this book, which brings a message to everyone who knows the pain of miscarriage and the desperate struggle to achieve the birth of a live, healthy baby in the face of frightening obstacles. This message is:

Take heart, for there is hope!

CONTENTS

Prologue: Fighting for your baby 5

1: True pregnancy tales of struggle, persistence, triumph 18

2: Dr David Barker's story 23

3: You're not alone! 41

4: Careers first...or babies first? 47

5: The making of a placenta 53

6: Fetus or baby? 63

7: The trimester myth 71

8: How your baby's weight can deceive you 81

9: Your womb's amazing capacity to recover 93

10: Miranda's choice 101

11: Your placenta as a computer system 111

12: Everything in your body matters to your baby 119

13: Things that can go wrong 127

14: Shelley's story 139

15: Testing, timing, prevention 147

16: The dreaded word (miscarriage) 161

17: The womb as a blood-clot bomb 173

18: Fran's story 189

19: Shocking truth of cardiovascular disease in women 201

20: The father's story 215

21: Fear of lawsuits; the politics of motherhood 225

22: Ruth's story 241

23: The price of an impaired placenta 259

24: The anatomy of a test 277

25: Multiple pregnancy 297

Epilogue: A Placenta Bill of Rights 305

Index 311

References 327

Prologue

FIGHTING FOR YOUR BABY

Of all human embryos conceived in the United States, 65% don't survive beyond four weeks. Of the survivors, one in four will miscarry.[1] Our nation should be ashamed of this disgraceful statistic which, at least for the foreseeable future, seems likely to increase, given that more women are becoming pregnant later in life than their mothers and grandmothers tended to do. In response to our horrifying pregnancy failure rate (which shouldn't be happening, for reasons I explain in this book), my mission is to bring you some good news. I am a perinatologist, also known as a maternal-fetal medicine physician, but I see myself chiefly as a placenta specialist. Over the decades, I've treated thousands of women who'd become convinced that they'd never successfully see their pregnancy to full term, let alone have a healthy baby. Today my office walls and files are full of photos of their thriving children.

The place where I happen to work is relevant to what I relate in this book. New York City is home to a great cross-section of America and, indeed, humanity. Whoever and wherever you, my reader, happen to be, I believe there are patients of mine, past and present, with whom you'd readily identify. They represent all levels of society, all faiths, all ethnicities. They are united by one desperate cry: "Please, help me have my baby."

This book is based on case after case of pregnancies which, after scary, agonizing complications, ended happily; surprisingly so, going by the US's shocking rate of high-risk pregnancy failure. I'm sharing with you here little-known facts from this trove of case histories that explain how these successful pregnancy outcomes came about. In particular, the following pages will open your eyes to the enormous importance of the hardest-working, most misunderstood and under-studied part of any pregnancy, the placenta, and its role in bringing about a successful birth, even against great odds. My clinical experiences, as a doctor specializing in high-risk pregnancies and pregnancy complications, have taught me remarkable things about the placenta. I believe this information will lift your spirits, giving you a new understanding of your body, your pregnancy outlook, and your capability to deal with the threats of miscarriage and high-risk pregnancy. This knowledge can empower you to take ownership of your pregnancy and teach you to communicate informedly with your medical team. You'll find out here, in plain, non-technical language, why you must demand that your placenta be monitored from conception. You'll also learn why you need to be prepared to fight from Day One to protect your pregnancy from miscarriage and other disasters related to the poverty of placenta knowledge that exists not only in the general public but also among doctors. My message is that if you're prepared to fight hard enough for your baby, you can reasonably aim to conquer more pregnancy setbacks and complications than you might have been led to believe is possible.

If your heart is set on having a baby despite pregnancy complications, you'll need all the determination you can muster, on several levels: physical, emotional, spiritual, intellectual. For decades, women have sat in my consulting rooms trembling with anxiety over whether they'd ever hear the birth cry of the child they so desperately wanted, and I've seen all too often how one of their hardest battles is an intellectual one: they've been worn out not just by false or misleading information but also by the sheer amount of information bombarding them. I've seen couples pounded into exhaustion by messages from every advertiser with a pregnancy-related product to hawk, not to mention avalanches of advice from friends, relatives, co-workers and acquaintances who well-intendedly pass on information both good and bad. Driven to their wits' end, would-be parents eventually reach the point of not wanting to hear and read another word; they feel they've been swamped by everything that's ever been said and written about pregnancy complications.

While working on this book, I asked myself many times whether I should add so much as a sentence to this deluge of opinions, allegations and factoids about pregnancy. Instead of writing, why not just continue my professional practice, helping one couple, baby, and mother at a time in my consulting rooms. After all, this has enabled me to see into the world thousands of healthy babies who otherwise might not have known good health or even life. So why write? These midnight thoughts loomed and boiled over me. The hammerings of doubt became my own passage through a storm, a personal journey I had to undergo in a process of writing and rewriting that took years. In the end, as with many authors, I found that sharing my experience through writing came to be a valuable oasis in my life and work, in the sense of an interlude enabling one to gather new strength. An oasis is a stage along the way, but there's also something of homecoming in it, or at least a promise of home which can be reached all the faster and better because you've found a quiet place from which to take new bearings. These feelings encouraged me to continue to write, heartened by my feeling that this book could become an oasis to women whom I wouldn't otherwise be able to reach through my medical practice. I came to think of my message in this book as one which could help such women gain new bearings of their own and a renewed sense of their pregnancy journey. The barrage of misinformation has made the already difficult pregnancy experiences of so many women disgracefully more nightmarish than necessary, and my hope and belief is that for many women and couples what I'm setting down here will be a refuge that will refresh them with new hope and direction in their quest for parenthood. Let me introduce you, then, to the kind of misinformation I want to help you fight off. A dangerous myth is widespread in our society. According to this myth, only when a pregnancy reaches a certain advanced point is it necessary to monitor the womb closely and be alert for serious problems.

If you're pregnant and have any reason to be concerned about the health of your baby, eject this myth from your mind at once. Pregnancy isn't a collection of neatly compartmented stages and events. It would certainly suit obstetricians if pregnancy were this convenient, as if accountants had designed it. Every process in the womb would take place in orderly separation from every other process. In such a charmingly simplified world, a doctor could in good conscience look at anything that happens in the womb without bothering about how it relates to anything else, the way financial bookkeepers separate one year's tax affairs from the next. But the womb doesn't work like this. It's a continuous, complex series of happenings which are interconnected in space and time. Every stage of your unborn baby's development has its own meaning, needs, risks and implications for what follows. To think that any stage, even the very earliest, can be safely disregarded is to court disaster. Understanding this can help you respond intelligently to the problems to which you and your baby may be vulnerable.

In pregnancy, as elsewhere, hard work pays off. Even with a deeply problematic medical history, you can have good reason to hope for a successful pregnancy if you're prepared to work with your womb, negotiating with it about its demands, all of which are reasonable. To do this effectively, you need to know as much as can find out about your own health. If any pregnancy complications are in your future, past or present, you must deal with them from the moment you know you're expecting. If possible, even before you become pregnant. You must also know how your womb works, and especially how your placenta works, even if this means abandoning some things you've previously read or been told. Consider this. By the 24th week of pregnancy, the placenta and fetus have reached roughly the same weight. Yet, halfway through the pregnancy, a healthy placenta will weigh more than the fetus. Now, this will happen only if early placenta growth has been healthy, and this "if" is tremendously important because during early placenta growth it's not that easy to know whether your placenta is developing as it should. If placenta development is poor for any reason in the first 24 weeks, it will be hard to detect this just by measuring the baby's weight with ultrasound. During this phase, the baby's needs and weight will seem OK even if the placenta is only half the size it should be. So the baby's weight can mislead you and your doctor. Because everyone's eyes are chiefly on the baby rather than the placenta, neither you nor your doctor would have any way to notice the placenta problem. It's common in high-risk pregnancies for complications to arise from this "placenta blind spot" phenomenon, which is the background to many pregnancy disasters. But when a placenta problem is detected early enough to fix it, the transformational effect on the pregnancy's health can be extraordinary. I've been at the bedsides of many mothers in whom this transformation has happened. Every time I'm as moved as if I'm witnessing it for the first time. It always awes me to see how the timely correction of a placenta problem can change the entire course of a pregnancy, pulling it from disaster and putting it back on track to a healthy birth. The placenta has an almost miraculous ability to save an endangered pregnancy. This amazing organ comes into being for the express purpose of supporting your pregnancy with immense physiological resources. To unlock this power, you have only to listen to what the placenta tells you.

So great is the placenta's power to help you, that it survives even death. When at the end of a delivery I look at the afterbirth (the placenta and related tissues which are expelled from a mother's body after the baby is born), I'm as moved as I am when the baby itself made its triumphant appearance. Just as the newborn quivers with a thousand stories waiting to be written, so the afterbirth palpitates with memories of the nine months or so preceding birth. If we examine the afterbirth, we find that even with its main work done, it can still offer us precious information about the health of the newborn for years to come. Often, however, the placenta is as sadly ignored after the pregnancy as it is during it.

For these reasons, even while this book seeks to help you reject dangerous myths which mystify pregnancy excessively, it's also aimed at helping you appreciate the genuinely mysterious aspects of this majestic process. It's here that some of the most inspiring reasons for hope are in reach for couples who desperately want a baby but are so battered by pregnancy failures, and by the unavailability of answers and solutions, that they feel nature is somehow conspiring against them, which is the opposite of the truth. In regard to pregnancy, your body is in fact a miracle of support and cooperation which asks only that you understand its ways. This has been shown to me again and again in the form of clinical experiences which have filled me with awe. The concept of awe has today been debased; people may tell you it is awesome that you can meet them for coffee, and once-rare scenes of genuinely awe-inspiring quality have become commonplace thanks to technologies which bring into easy reach countless images of natural wonder, from the bottom of the sea to scenes of other worlds. But nothing is a more fitting object of awe than childbirth and pregnancy. A full appreciation of this is strangely absent from our culture, which tends rather to minimize the extraordinary aspects of pregnancy and make them as ordinary as possible, perhaps because this helps powerful institutions like insurance companies minimize their responsibility for pregnancy success.

Despite all the decades I have practiced as a maternal-fetal medicine specialist I never cease to come out of the delivery room with the same awe that I felt when I delivered newborns for the very first time, except that now my awe is all the richer and more layered and nuanced because of my long experience with complicated pregnancies, which has made me more aware than ever of the vast mystery, powers and still-to-be-understood attributes of the womb, and especially the placenta. Every man, woman, girl and boy who walks the earth is the product of what happened within a placenta. This fleshy organ, humbly keeping out of sight with a mother's body and ceding the spotlight to the fetus and then the baby that it so faithfully serves, is the close companion of each one of us for some nine months before at last we bid farewell to the womb. We need to acquire a new respect, even reverence, for this majestic phenomenon.

On the other hand, the need to de-mystify pregnancy failure arises because doctors all too often treat events like miscarriage as if they're inexplicable. While medical science has much yet to learn, we already know quite a bit about why many pregnancies end badly. Unfortunately, the medical establishment isn't geared to encourage the sharing of much of this information among doctors, let alone with patients. The culture of professional specialization actually discourages or at least greatly slows down the sharing of knowledge between one specialty and another. Also, while scientifically trained people like doctors are widely believed to be in the forefront of knowledge, they often lag surprisingly far behind knowledge growth because of the bureaucratic way their profession "certifies" knowledge, legitimizing it as "official" only long after it's been shown to be valid and even put extensively into practical use.

Yet another factor in the mystification of events like miscarriage is the great power of health insurance companies. If a search for a medical explanation requires the insurer to pay for investigative work, the doctor will generally be "discouraged" from pursuing it. It's cheaper to attribute a miscarriage to bad luck and "nature's way." Contrary to this commercially convenient non-explanation, placenta science can frequently explain the causes of poor pregnancy outcomes in ways that can help put a mother on a better pregnancy path. And here's the irony: insurers and compliant, complacent doctors don't have to invent depressing mystery to superimpose on pregnancy because there's more than enough genuine mystery about it, and far from being discouraging, the authentically mysterious aspects of pregnancy tend to offer reasons for optimism rather than feeling helpless and retreating into passive acceptance.

These grounds for pregnancy optimism (at least as I express them) don't currently form part of conventional pregnancy care philosophy. This is why I've said that, as a mother, you need to take ownership of your pregnancy. This may sound strange. You'd think the desire for a healthy pregnancy is so strong that no woman could possibly lose ownership of her pregnancy. Yet many do exactly that. They surrender their pregnancy to despair, to myths and misinformation, to the unchallenged habits of the medical establishment, including practices imposed by insurance companies for their profit and financial convenience.

In order to take ownership of your pregnancy, you'll need to act on the information I provide in this book. And I must make it clear that, although this information comes largely from the case files of two New York clinics in which I've worked for the past several decades and amassed my clinical knowledge, this doesn't mean you should necessarily seek treatment at these clinics. If you're experiencing pregnancy complications or expect to have to deal with them, I urge you to use the information in these pages to help yourself as best as you can in the area where you live. Use what you learn here as a guide to ask your doctor the right questions, insist on the right treatments, and take the steps that placenta knowledge shows to be necessary for a successful full-term pregnancy. This book is, in fact, intended as a guide to you in building your relationship with your doctor. Nothing in these pages can substitute for a consultation with a physician whom you choose and trust. Even though I'm a physician specializing in maternal-fetal medicine, the fact that I've written a book which you have decided to read doesn't make me your doctor, or enable me to give you medical advice about your pregnancy or other health issues. I'd be able to offer you personal medical advice only if I were first to examine you. But regardless of who examines you and is called upon to advise you on your pregnancy, and help you manage it, you need to take ownership of your pregnancy and not be a passive patient. Respect your doctor but be proactive. Assert your rights and be unafraid to question procedures which happen to be preferred by insurance companies or other institutions. Remember, it's your body and your baby.

From time to time in this book, scary messages may seem to alternate confusingly with optimistic ones. One moment, I'm talking about horrifying dangers to your pregnancy, while the next moment, I talk about your placenta's amazing resilience and the significant scope that exists for you to save your baby from disaster. These sets of messages aren't contradictory, though; both the scary messages and the optimistic ones are true. The key to their compatibility is the question of timing that I'll keep stressing. If you take timely action to correct problems in any high-risk pregnancy, you can be assured that there is a highly realistic hope for a good outcome. This statement is grounded in firm clinical knowledge and experience, based on not dozens or hundreds but thousands of stories of complicated pregnancies which have been brought to a successful fruition, generally against great odds if we go by the high-risk pregnancy failure rate prevailing in our society.

I feel overwhelming, humble gratitude to my many patients through the years whose cases have enabled me to bring you such strongly felt assurance and hope, derived not from theoretical conviction but from clinical experience. Time after time, I have put a healthy newborn into the waiting arms of a mother who'd been led to believe, by someone along her pregnancy journey, that this would not happen, or at least that it was highly unlikely. No sight in the world can match such a mother's reaction when she touches her baby for the first time and hears it demand its rightful attention with the indignant authority that only a baby can project. This cry, which has been heard down all the ages, is the voice of life itself, and even the most devoutly secular persons feel in their bones that there is in this imperative sound something that can only be called sacred. This is all the more clear and eloquent when one knows that mother and baby have endured and conquered potentially fatal obstacles to get to this point.

I'm a doctor, not a miracle worker. Too often patients with complicated pregnancies have come to me far too late, with their placenta or its supporting physiology so compromised by inadequate treatments based on poor placenta knowledge that I couldn't save that pregnancy, even though I may have been able to offer hope for the next one. Even after thousands of patients, it never gets easier to sit down with a couple who, having placed all their hopes in the fragile life beneath the bump, must now hear that the climax of pregnancy will not be the greeting cry of birth but that awful silence that's more oppressive than any other: the stillness of unachieved life. And it makes this suffering immeasurably deeper to know that if only placenta science had been properly applied soon enough, the outcome would likely have been a different and joyful one. I have had too many of these heartbreaking conversations, followed by solitary anguishing over the shortcomings of an insurance-controlled medical establishment. As I've contemplated the unlived child lives that should have filled the homes of my bereft patients, I've realized the emptiness and unwisdom of asking, even as I compulsively felt myself asking: what might this unborn child have become? It is out of my rebellion against my having had to think these thoughts so many times that I embark on my mission in this book, which is to tell women (and men, who I have found to be as capable of emotional investment in pregnancy as women) that there isn't just hope but also clinical knowledge that can justify that hope, with only the proviso that time is an unbending ruler of all things and that even the womb's overwhelming will to life must bow to its impositions. Thus, while there's more hope for a way out of complicated pregnancies than most people realize, there's also such a thing as Too Late. So to all those who read this book with a successful birth in mind, especially against a background of past or present pregnancy complications, I write with a sense of impassioned urgency.

It's common for books about complicated matters to be written in a linear style, with the author presenting one set of facts or train of thought and then leaving it behind to move on to the next one. I'm not following this conventional method here, though. To my mind, just about everything I have to tell you is connected with other things you need to know, because with pregnancy problems, just about everything is intimately connected with everything else: if you separate facts too much for convenience, you distort them. This book is therefore written in a non-linear style. After I tell you something, I won't regard that subject as finished and done. I'll come back to it later, usually from a different angle. This method, I believe, will give you a richer understanding than would otherwise have been possible. It also has the advantage of periodically reminding you of what you read earlier, and the facts of pregnancy can be so complex that I think you'll find this helpful.

Chapter 1

TRUE PREGNANCY STORIES OF STRUGGLE, PERSISTENCE ... AND TRIUMPH

To illustrate some of the information I'm sharing with you I'm going to tell you true stories about some of my patients. To protect their privacy, I'm changing names and disguising some details, but the essential events of the stories are exactly as I describe.

I'm also going to tell you something of my own story as a specialist in high-risk pregnancies and pregnancy complications. Because my experiences with my patients have taught me much that I wasn't taught in medical school, I believe it's not enough for me simply to tell you the medical facts. I want you to know how I encountered these facts in my consulting rooms, and how they've shaped my whole understanding of pregnancy. I therefore have to give you some sense of myself, my life and my reflections on my career as a high-risk pregnancy doctor.

In addition, I'm going to tell you the story of pregnancy itself: about how vulnerable a human fetus is, how much respect its needs must receive, and how and why that hugely underestimated marvel of biology, your placenta, is vital to these needs. And yet another story I'll tell you is how your amazing system of natural health maintenance and self-regulation, evolved over eons, enables pregnancies to happen, to be sustained over long months of staggeringly complex development, and to bring forth healthy babies.

To call the womb astonishing is a vast understatement. It encompasses mechanisms which respond to crises and fine-tune fetal well-being in a subtle process of ongoing interaction between the brain, body chemistry, nervous system, blood circulation and numerous other physiological phenomena. The best way to help your unborn baby is to work with this ongoing fetal health-maintenance process, diligently and with humility. Many doctors, I suspect, fail to achieve optimal cooperation with the natural power of a woman's body because of insufficient humility in the face of this fetal system's extraordinariness. For example:

Some years ago, I was called on to examine an 18-week fetus with swelling behind the neck that led in a week to mild hydrops (a fluid accumulation illness). Genes and body structure were normal, but as its blood group was incompatible with its mother's, the fetus was severely anemic; i.e. its blood lacked key components. It was given an intrauterine blood transfusion over 15 minutes. Minutes later, one of the heart chambers (the right ventricle) became enlarged and stopped contracting for a few seconds. An immediate Doppler examination (more about this technology later) showed a heart valve malfunction and abnormal blood flow in two major veins, the ductus venosus and umbilical vein. By all appearances, the fetus was dying. There were two possible causes: the anemia or the transfusion, which may have strained the heart's functionality.

What happened next flabbergasted us. The ductus venosus vein takes oxygenated blood from the placenta to another important vein (the inferior vena cava) and a heart chamber called the right atrium. Now, the ductus does this only in the womb: after birth it loses its blood-carrying function. It's one of three blood vessels called "shunts" which temporarily carry fetal blood while the fetus is developing. These shunts are vital routes for supplying oxygen-enriched blood to the fetal brain. None of this prepared us for what we saw. As we watched, the blood in the ductus venosus reversed direction and flowed backward towards the placenta from which it had come, allowing it to offload the strain. A few minutes later, the heart function normalized.

It was unheard of for blood in the ductus venosus to reverse direction. Yet we not only saw this happen but recorded it with Doppler technology. We also then saw the heart recover from its crisis almost immediately. The clinical team members couldn't say for sure, then or later, whether the recovery and the reversal were connected, and, if so, how, but from what we know about the placenta's ability to store excess blood, it makes sense to theorize that this was a natural physiological mechanism that somehow saved the fetus's life. Whatever the exact explanation might one day turn out to be, two points stand out. First, several colleagues and I undoubtedly witnessed a hard-to-explain recovery from the apparent brink of fetal death after a blood flow reversal which was contrary to available medical knowledge. Second, when my colleagues and I tried to share our observations of this remarkable event, we had great difficulty getting other doctors to believe us! A medical journal told us, with a tone of ridicule, that we must have imagined it, as such reversal was impossible. Why? Because it had never been reported before. So we went to another journal and got a similar response. Exasperated, we gave up our publishing effort. Then, some two years later, at a scientific convention, doctors unconnected with my group presented not one but two reports of blood flow reversal in the ductus! Encouraged, we submitted our report again. This time it was published.[2]

This true story shows that pregnancy contains wonders literally beyond imagination, confounding learned doctors whose closed minds dismiss anything outside their comfort zones. Mothers and babies are badly let down by such closed minds, because many true stories attest to the astonishing things that are possible in a woman's body when the struggle for fetal life is at stake. Even the apparently bleakest pregnancy outlooks can end well, especially if we adopt a new attitude toward the placenta, whose function is to use powerful biological processes, evolved over immensities of time, to achieve one goal: the successful birth of a healthy baby. When I speak of taking ownership of your pregnancy, one of the things I mean is, that as a mother you have to be prepared to take responsibility for championing a new level of respect for these processes within you, and doing this means fighting the kind of closed mind I've just described. Those patients of mine who've achieved some of the most impressive victories over pregnancy complications have tended to have a tremendous sense of personal responsibility for the happenings inside them and for how they communicated with doctors about these things. Such personal responsibility can seem frightening, but it becomes less so when you start to realize the extent of the powers at work in the womb. This will arm you to think about your womb outside the limits of conventional pregnancy narratives. I can't emphasize too strongly how important it is for you to burst through these limits of conventional pregnancy thought. Although I'm a fully credentialed, board-certified maternal-fetal medicine specialist now in my 4th decade of clinical practice in New York, a good deal of my success in beating the US's pregnancy failure rate is due to my having learned to think against many prevailing pregnancy beliefs of not only the general public but also the medical establishment.

Please understand: I'm not saying you must disrespect physicians. Being one myself, I can tell you with confidence how hard it is to become a licensed medical practitioner. However, it's just human nature that great learning makes it easy to overestimate the amount we've learned, and to underestimate or trivialize the extent of our ignorance. The best way to approach this is by keeping in mind that doctors, like everyone else, have both fallibility and feelings. When you challenge your doctor's advice, always do so respectfully and with calm explanation.

And now I want to tell you a story about a patient of mine I'll call Mary.

~

Mary's experience offers an excellent introduction to the placenta's power, as well as to the interconnectedness that I described earlier as a feature of pregnancy knowledge. In traditional fiction, stories have a beginning, a middle and an end. In pregnancy, things aren't that neat. Mothers can find themselves suddenly caught up in circumstances that seem to have descended on them from nowhere. This is what happened to Mary. She mistakenly thought that with two intensively managed pregnancies behind her, nothing could go wrong with her third. But this pregnancy turned out to involve a crisis, a mystery, and a medical detective story that illuminates the extraordinary relationship existing between the placenta and an unborn baby's brain.

One day, Mary found herself experiencing something so

bizarre that she thought this must be what an out-of-the-body experience felt like. It left her dazed, frightened, and confused. Just a short while earlier, everything had seemed to be going well. She'd been so closely monitored at every step of the way in both of her first two pregnancies that it seemed everything about her body, including every potential pregnancy risk factor, had been identified and charted in detail. In view of this, it seemed reasonable to suppose that all aspects of her latest pregnancy must be utterly under control. But, just a few days ago, it had been learned that the umbilical cord had become wrapped around her baby's neck. When this happens, most babies suffer no harm, but in some cases a fetal movement can cause compression of the umbilical vessels, reducing the baby's oxygen supply. In severe cases, this can cause fetal brain damage and even death. Mary therefore understood when she was told it was now necessary to monitor not only the baby's condition but also the blood flow in the umbilical cord, so as to identify any compression of the umbilical vein or umbilical artery.

Nevertheless, everything had seemed to be under control. In fact, she'd come to her doctor today for a relatively routine examination. But almost immediately alarm bells went off. Mary suddenly found herself in the middle of a whirl of medical discussions being conducted around her and over her with a sense of fearful urgency. Then she heard her baby must be delivered immediately! She wasn't ready for this, emotionally or any other way, yet here she was, being prepped for an emergency cesarean section. In this hubbub, her thoughts flew in many directions including a rush of memories of everything that had led to this moment.

In each of Mary's three pregnancies, conception had been

easy, despite the fact that she'd been diagnosed before her first pregnancy as having a bifurcated (or bicornuate) uterus, i.e. one that was abnormally divided in two sections. This abnormality can prevent natural conception, and once conception is achieved, it can lead to premature birth. In Mary's case neither occurred. How, then, had she got to what was happening to her today? As she lay quivering in the operating theater, her mind traveled back four years.

~

With her first pregnancy, she'd been referred to a specialist because tests showed she'd inherited a mild form of a blood-clotting disease, thrombophilia. This didn't cause much concern, though, because it was a well-known disorder that could be effectively managed if diagnosed in good time, as was the case here. So no one expected any unpleasant surprises. Mary was examined fortnightly and given an anticoagulant medication to inject into her abdomen twice daily. Things went well for some 16 weeks. Then a routine ultrasound exam revealed damage to the placenta. Fetal blood flow wasn't good, so the baby's growth had slowed. But what was causing this problem? Mild thrombophilia couldn't be responsible for this much harm. A hunt for a deeper cause began.

Could the baby's father, Jim, have thrombophilia too? He was tested, and sure enough, he had 3 genetic mutations linked to thrombophilia. This compounded the effect of Mary's mild case of the disease ... and it meant the baby, too, had thrombophilia. Mary's blood-thinning medication was increased. The usual dose is 40 milligrams once daily and in difficult cases twice daily, but Mary took 60 milligrams in the morning and 40 in the evening. With this aggressive treatment, the baby's growth rate improved and the placenta stabilized. But by 24 weeks, it looked like there was no way to reverse the damage. All that could be aimed for was to arrest the thrombophilia-induced decline and avoid further deterioration until the pregnancy reached at least 32 weeks, when the baby could be delivered with relative safety.

In the 31st week, Mary was at work when she suddenly started bleeding. She phoned her doctor, who told her to go to the hospital immediately. She later recalled: "I'd had a steroid injection the night before to promote the baby's lung maturity because there was a possibility this baby might be born prematurely. I thought that the bleeding might be a side effect from that shot. Even though I was told many times that there weren't side effects, I still couldn't wrap my mind around why this was happening. I was told to go directly to labor and delivery and asked to fill out paperwork for admittance, but after the nurse handed me the documents and took a look at the shape I was in, she said: *Forget filling out the paper. Let's get you hooked up to a monitor.* I realized then how much blood I'd lost and how pale I was. This was not a side effect. I remember thinking: *Who doesn't fill out paperwork to get admitted to a hospital? People who are in serious trouble!* And I started to cry. The nurse was so nice. She calmed me down, hooked me up to the monitor, and when we heard the baby's heart rate, her look of relief was probably the same as mine. I knew she had a better understanding of what was happening than I did and I was so grateful for her kindness. But I had no idea what we were in for."

Doctors started to come in to assess the situation, starting with the youngest resident physician. On seeing the extent of Mary's bleeding she consulted a more senior resident, who went for help to the most senior resident, who decided to call in the top attending physician responsible for delivery that night. As the gravity of

Mary's condition became more apparent, Mary's husband Jim arrived and the rest of her family started showing up. The fear on their faces frightened her more than anything the doctors said.

Mary was hospitalized on a Thursday. She was put under continuous electronic fetal monitoring and given an ultrasound exam every two days to assess fetal and placenta blood flow. When Tuesday came, something new showed up: high blood flow resistance in the uterine artery. This abnormality can signal impending placenta abruptio, when the placenta comes loose from the uterus wall, causing severe bleeding and fetal asphyxia (deprivation of oxygen). This prompted a decision to deliver immediately. "I was scared and nervous about the baby being born so early," Mary said later. "But still I felt everything would be OK. We'd just seen the baby on the sonogram and she looked good." She was taken back to her hospital room feeling reassured. But about ten minutes later she began bleeding again. "This time it was different. There was a lot more blood, and it wouldn't stop. Doctors and nurses came running into the room. It was the most frightening experience of my life. I could see the worry in their eyes. Some of the nurses were crying with me. I was in shock. After everything we had gone through, we might lose the baby now? We'd just seen the heartbeat on the sonogram."

In the labor and delivery room, Mary's placenta did indeed detach abruptly from her uterus. Fortunately the clear warnings had prepared the medical team for this. In Mary's words: "Everything happened so fast. I was hysterical. They rushed me into an operating room for an emergency C-section. I was given general anesthesia because there was no time for an epidural. I was completely out during the delivery." Unconscious when her daughter Lily arrived (small but otherwise in excellent condition),

Mary reflected afterwards: "I still can't believe how close we came to losing her and how lucky we are that we have such a happy and healthy little girl."

But that was just the beginning.

Because Lily had survived only because of intensive placenta monitoring, Mary's next pregnancy was closely and frequently monitored from the outset, with steps to pre-empt her known medical issues. This worked. Mary and Jim welcomed a healthy son, Steve, after a full-term pregnancy without incident. Based on this experience, it seemed Mary was now home free with no more unknowns lying in wait. Not so! When Mary conceived a third time, it did at first look like everything her doctors had learned about her body, along with the now established policy of intensive, pre-emptive management, was paying off. Things went well. Then, 12 weeks into the pregnancy, something strange happened to Mary's placenta. More precisely, to her chorionic villi (finger-shaped protuberances that project from the chorion, a membrane around unborn babies), which transfer oxygen and food from the mother's blood to the baby's. (Bear with me; I'll explain more about pregnancy physiology in a little while.) Mary's villi stopped doing their job properly, so her baby stopped receiving all the oxygen and nutrients it needed for continued healthy growth.

This was puzzling, because in all the copious data about Mary that had by now been amassed there was no hint that something would go wrong with her chorionic villi. The thrombophilia couldn't be blamed because it was under control with medication. So more tests were done. These revealed a new, previously unsuspected culprit: Mary's own immune system. This system is the body's army. It's a network of processes whose task is to protect you against any outside element that might invade you and make you ill. But sometimes it malfunctions, losing the ability to distinguish between friend and foe. It then behaves like a rogue army, attacking the very tissues and cells it's supposed to defend. Mary's body was attacking part of itself. Specifically her placenta. This was the first time she'd shown any sign of such a disorder, which can take various forms. In this case what was happening was that a group of her "soldier cells," with the colorful but accurate name of Natural Killer or NK cells, were on the rampage, running amok against her placenta tissues which they were mistakenly perceiving as invasive matter. To counteract these out-of-control cells, Mary was started on two-weekly lipid (fat) emulsion infusions, which are known to curb rogue NK activity. This did the trick: her villi recovered and the pregnancy settled down again; everyone breathed a sigh of relief. Then, during a regular check-up at 34 weeks, another problem was discovered.

Mary's baby was found to be undergoing a phenomenon called brain sparing.[3,4] This is one of the most remarkable protective processes in pregnancy. When, for any reason, the placenta doesn't supply enough oxygen-rich blood, the fetus starts giving first priority of blood supply to its most important organs: the brain, heart and adrenal glands. (The brain is the body's control center; the heart governs the body's nutrient delivery system through the blood, and if the heart stops beating no blood, and thus no food or oxygen, will go anywhere; the adrenal glands produce hormones, signaling chemicals that tell organs what to do and when.)

This emergency step of "rationing" oxygen comes at a high price. In prioritizing the brain, heart and adrenals to receive most of the oxygen and nutrients which are in short supply, the fetal circulation robs some parts of the body to look after others. An unborn baby can cope with this only up to a point. If the problem that triggered the brain sparing is fixed before a critical point is reached, so that normal oxygenation and nutrition are restored in time throughout the baby's body, fine. But if brain sparing lasts too long, the oxygen-deprived parts of the baby, including the liver, kidneys and muscles, can be irreparably damaged. Brain sparing is therefore not something the body does lightly. When doctors see it, they know the placenta's in big trouble.

Mary could sense the deep anxiety of her medical team. "I knew as soon as the technician started the scan that there was a serious issue," she said later. "She kept running the same tests over and over again and I could tell by her face that she was concerned. She left the room to get the doctor. When he came in he also looked concerned and began to run the scans again. After a few minutes he stopped and said we needed to have the baby today." It all happened so fast that although the brain sparing was explained to Mary, the details flew past her and she went into the delivery theater still under the impression that the rush was due to the umbilical cord being wrapped around the baby's neck. Although the cord wasn't the reason, it did have some effect: Mary's new daughter, Joan, was born with a mild breathing problem. (She recovered from this in the intensive care unit.) But it was the brain sparing that had been pivotal in saving Joan's life. As Mary has put it: "We were lucky to get her out when we did."

Throughout her three pregnancies Mary was attended by several doctors. Each had an important role in seeing her babies through. Mine included discovering that the brain sparing was under way. Mary's then obstetrician-gynecologist graciously telephoned me afterwards, putting me on speaker so he and Mary could both share their joy that this diagnosis was made in time to make a crucial difference which valuably serves, to this day, as an example of the womb's magnificent architecture and processes.

But there's more. At the time, no one realized just how close to death baby Joan had been before her crisis delivery. Although the brain sparing had been recognized in time to save her, there was, once again, bewilderment about exactly what had triggered it. The usual cause of brain sparing, you see, is placenta damage. Yet Mary's placenta looked fine. You'll remember that her immune system problem had been dealt with. So why should her baby's body have initiated brain sparing? This process is essentially a healthy baby's way of reacting to an increasingly hostile uterine environment, and essentially saying: "Get me out of here!"

Then a pattern of clues started forming.

First, the obstetrician who delivered Joan reported having noticed, during the delivery, that one of the umbilical arteries was damaged, and possibly clotted despite Mary's anti-clotting medication. (By lowering the risk of maternal clotting, this medicine protects the baby from the ill effects of clots forming in the mother's bloodstream. The medicine doesn't penetrate into the baby's bloodstream and so can't protect against clots forming there. The baby itself can trigger a clot by, for example, lodging its foot against the umbilical cord.)

The second clue arose from my habit of examining the placenta and umbilical cord of all my patients after delivery. Sometimes other experts help me learn more about what this afterbirth can tell us about the completed pregnancy. Working together, maternal-fetal medicine specialists like myself, placenta pathologists and others form laboratory detective teams that often coax postpartum tissues into revealing unsuspected answers to puzzling questions, much as police scientists solve mysteries by studying apparently trivial clues from crime scenes. About a week or two after Joan was born, I received a visit from a pathologist I'd consulted about Mary's afterbirth. She brought with her a sample of Joan's umbilical cord. Her findings were disturbing: she'd learned that the cord had indeed contained a clot, so big that it had incapacitated one of the two umbilical arteries. Laboratory analysis of the clotted umbilical artery suggested that the initial clot formation was almost seven days old. Such findings are commonly associated with fetal death. As usual, though, the paperwork requesting the pathology report didn't indicate whether or not the baby had survived. From the available evidence, the pathologist thought she was examining tissues from a pregnancy in which the baby had died seven days before we delivered Joan ... alive and healthy.

The pathologist's findings thus solved a puzzle but posed a new one. The solved puzzle was why the brain sparing had occurred despite Mary's healthy, closely monitored placenta. It was due not to placenta insufficiency (brain sparing's most common trigger), but to the sudden clotting. Moreover, although the clotting might have been worsened by the thrombophilia, the most likely initial and dominant cause was the entanglement of the umbilical cord -- an unpredictable accident in the random changes of fetal position. This, then, prompted the new mystery: how did baby Joan survive as long as she did despite oxygen deprivation which, according to all the available scientific evidence, should have been fatal?

There seems to be only one answer, and although physicians aren't supposed to attribute desires to natural processes, and although the tissues of the body outside the brain possess no consciousness and thus no will in any scientifically conventional sense, I don't mind putting it this way: on a level that is meaningful despite our present inability to express its meaning in scientific language, Mary's body was just determined that Joan must live.

~

In addition to the humbling lesson that this case teaches us about the profound ability of even the weakest organism to fight for life, it has several more things to tell us. Mary's babies were all born to the same mother, yet each baby had a different pregnancy story. Every pregnancy is ultimately unique. Then, there's a lesson here about the limits of human prediction. Doctors often like to inspire confidence by pretending, I believe, to know more than they do. Of course they need to project a reassuring authority, but when it's taken too far it can be a great mistake. Despite the wealth of information that had been built up due to Mary's close monitoring, there was no way, at least with available medical knowledge, to predict either the NK cell upsurge or the umbilical cord accident, any more than there was to predict baby Joan's astonishing ability to survive the undetected clot against all scientifically known odds. (It was eventually concluded that Mary's cord clot had formed not suddenly but gradually over at least seven days, following injury or mild prolonged compression, and Joan had slowly adapted to survive.)

Mary's case also shows that despite our limited abilities to anticipate womb events, intensive and sustained monitoring do pay off for women with known pregnancy problems. If Mary hadn't been monitored so closely, the brain sparing would likely not have been recognized in time to take the emergency action that saved Joan's life. Finally, Mary's story is an excellent introduction to the marvels of the lifeline of the unborn: the placenta. Which brings me to the story of a man who pioneered the modern era of placenta knowledge. Learning a bit about him will help you to understand your own placenta.

Chapter 2

DR DAVID BARKER'S STORY

The human body is an intricate weave of biological and chemical systems: a mini-universe of worlds within worlds, encompassing a spectacular diversity of structures that range from the microscopic to those visible to the naked eye. Among all these structures, the placenta is unique. This one organ is the center of every woman's pregnancy quest and of everything that your childbearing experience will mean for the health and future of your baby. Not only during pregnancy, but long after you give birth.

As the link between your fetus and the wall of your uterus, your placenta holds the key to the kinds of miscarriages to which you may be vulnerable, if any. Your placenta's health will be crucial in deciding whether or not you'll see your pregnancy through.

For the months in which your unborn baby lives in you, your placenta must feed it, channeling nutrients to it from your own bloodstream, sharing your oxygen with it, and removing waste material that would otherwise accumulate harmfully. In a healthy pregnancy, your placenta will do all this in a meticulously measured manner, giving your baby exactly what it needs with a precision akin to that of a sophisticated computer. And yet, amazingly, not only to the general public but also to most physicians, the placenta today remains the least-understood part of the reproductive process. General recognition of the placenta's importance is so relatively recent that on October 4, 2010, the editors of Time magazine featured it as their cover news story, with the headline: "How the first nine months shape the rest of your life: the new science of fetal origins."

A strange aspect of this dramatic report was that while it was indeed news to many people, including most doctors, there was also a sense in which it wasn't news at all. It dated back to 1992, when a physician, Dr David Barker, published a scientific article showing for the first time that babies born underweight were at greater risk of developing coronary heart disease as adults. In 1995, BMJ, the official journal of the British Medical Association, named this finding the Barker Hypothesis. Since then it's become widely accepted that our adult health is significantly affected by what happened to us in the womb. Our pre-birth experiences affect our adult risk of, e.g., heart disease, obesity, cancer, hypertension and type 2 diabetes.[5-8]

Barker's Hypothesis is also known as the Fetal Programming Hypothesis. This word choice has both negative and positive connotations. The negative is that we see computers as programmed to function in certain ways and no others. We think of robots as having no choice. Associating pregnancy with this lack of alternatives is problematic because it suggests pregnancy outcomes are at the mercy of forces wholly beyond our influence, which isn't true. On the other hand, the programming analogy has a valuable connotation in that computers can be re-programmed, and so, to a certain extent, can your body's responses to pregnancy. Realizing this creates a significantly (and justifiably) more optimistic view of pregnancy. Certainly, nature places constraints on us. But when we cooperate with nature, it rewards us by giving us a say in how things turn out. By respecting nature and seeking to understand its workings through a combination of science and common sense, we become empowered to help program (or reprogram) the way natural processes unfold. For example, many people assume our genes pretty much irrevocably shape what happens to us, but Barker's research led him to conclude that this is not quite true. By understanding how your pregnancy "programs" your baby's health, before birth and after it, you can, in fact, participate in that programming.

Barker, who died in 2013, was a British medical scientist and physician who trained at two leading hospitals, Guy's Hospital, in London, and the Queen Elizabeth Centre, in Birmingham. He taught medicine in Britain and Africa before becoming a professor of clinical science at the University of Southampton. From 2003, he also served as a professor in America, at Oregon Health & Science University, in Portland, Oregon. His work has come to be widely accepted. According to Professor Eileen Kennedy, of the Friedman School of Nutrition Science and Policy at Tufts University, in Medford, Massachusetts, Barker's research has been "ground- breaking" and has "irrevocably influenced" medical thinking. Dr Ricardo Uauy, former president of the International Union of Nutritional Sciences, has stated that Barker's research "gives us the unique opportunity to re-examine the role of nutrition throughout life, and place the emphasis where it really makes a difference, in early life. Good nutrition begins in the womb. It is time for this novel insight to make it into policy and practice."

Dr Kent Thornburg, director of the Heart Research Center at Oregon Health and Science University, has commented: "History will show that David Barker's discoveries changed the face of medicine." These opinions of Barker's work were confirmed in his lifetime by his receipt of major scientific prizes, including medals from Britain's Royal Society and Royal College of Physicians. From all this you would think that Barker's work has revolutionized how doctors manage pregnancy. But not so. Full appreciation of his ideas has tended to be limited to a relatively specialized research community. In the wider medical community the recognition has been far smaller, and a deep understanding of the implications has been smaller still.

One of the most important things about Barker's research is that he wasn't just a doctor of medicine or even primarily a pregnancy specialist. He was an epidemiologist. Epidemiology is the science of the causes of disease. In 2011 he was awarded the world's top prize in this field, the Richard Doll Prize. This matters to your pregnancy because it means Barker's chief aim was to understand the causes of illness throughout adult life. This led him to investigate the connections between the illnesses that afflict us in the womb and those we develop in adulthood. As a result, he found it necessary to study what can go wrong in the womb, and why.

Why has Barker's groundbreaking research become "news" only relatively recently? One reason is that scientific establishments are rightly skeptical of new findings and theories. Another reason is that the medical profession, in particular, likes its established habits. Science is widely thought of as being open to constant change, but medical professionals tend to be quite conservative.

Barker first theorized that adult diseases could originate

in the womb when he noticed a strong link between low birthweight and increased risk for adult cardiovascular disease. When he first presented his data, he was jeered because his conclusions contradicted most physicians' beliefs. Resistance wasn't universal, though. Some doctors were excited because their own clinical work was consistent with Barker's findings. My own experiences had compelled me to think along lines similar to Barker's conclusions, so much so that by 1993, the year after he published his major paper, I decided it was imperative to publish a book in non-technical language so I could share my own findings with readers outside the medical profession, especially women facing pregnancy challenges. For a long time, though, I fully expected Barker's work to cause such an explosion of education about womb health, especially regarding the placenta, that a book by me would be unnecessary. But the spreading of placenta knowledge didn't happen. The information I'm presenting in this book is as badly needed now as it was in 1993, if not more so.

I myself first learned about the placenta in 1974. I was a 4th-year medical student at Alexandra Hospital in Athens, Greece. Although my role model was a successful obstetrician (my uncle Zachary), I'd never thought of becoming one. But when I did my required course in obstetrics and gynecology, I found that my medical textbook's 350 pages or so included a single page on the placenta. I was stunned and my life changed. This seemed very wrong. I became obsessed with learning about the placenta. My thoughts of a general surgery career faded. Obstetrics and gynecology took over my mind. (In a sense, it wasn't a big change because obstetricians and gynecologists have to be good surgeons in their specialty.)

On coming to America, I found that placenta studies were

expanding rapidly, yet information wasn't being applied directly to clinical practice. Then, in the 1980s, a new field, maternal-fetal medicine, began emerging. I was elated to be one of the first doctors trained to practice in what was then a cutting-edge discipline. By 1993, when the idea of this book took root, I was at York Hospital, Pennsylvania, directing the division that trained University of Pennsylvania medical students and obstetrical residents in maternal-fetal medicine. My mission was to help these trainee physicians understand that an obstetrician's job isn't just to deliver babies but to manage pregnancy as a window on the baby's (and mother's) future health. In keeping with Barker's work, I was convinced that if we took into account how womb events could shape adult life, this same information must also shed light on things that go wrong in the womb. My clinical work has overwhelmingly confirmed this conclusion.

As a result of this philosophy, my obstetrical group developed a new description of the aims of obstetric care, seeing pregnancy as a defining moment not only in the mother's life but, even more so, in the life of the fetus, of the person that the fetus would become, and of the entire chain of events which connected all of these in a total and unified physiological reality. Using the limited knowledge of the placenta and fetal development that then existed (long before the accumulation of research that Time Magazine would report in 2010), my group concluded that the fetus's nine months or so of life inside the mother's uterus was the most important time in any person's life, and that it was during these crucial months of pregnancy that the fetus and placenta together developed the foundation of childhood and adult heath. Thus, in our effort to better define the obstetrician's relationship with the pregnant mother, our clinical group concluded back in

1993 that the obstetric mission should be to protect not only the mother from pregnancy-related complications but also the fetus, helping it realize its genetic potential within the womb, then as a newborn baby, as a child, and finally as an adult. This idea, seeing womb events as the single most crucial factor in both the short-term success of the pregnancy and the lifelong health of the human being that the fetus would become, continued to govern my work after I became chief of Maternal-Fetal Medicine in the Department of Obstetrics and Gynecology at Brooklyn Hospital Center, New York, in 1994, and then the head of Kofinas Perinatal, the clinic I established in New York in 2000.

A key difference between Barker and myself was that he approached womb knowledge as an epidemiologist, seeking causes of adult illness, whereas my aim as a clinician was to make every woman's pregnancy as successful as possible for both her and her baby. The center of my work thus became the experiences of all the women who've chosen to entrust their pregnancy problems to me. This has made me deeply aware that successful pregnancy management isn't only physiological; it's also about overcoming psychological barriers. There isn't just a failure to appreciate the importance of the placenta. There are also misleading impressions of the ease of pregnancy. Even as more couples struggle to have a baby, so media narratives continue to circulate stereotypes of women becoming pregnant without effort or intention, and with a bouncing baby arriving nine months later, assuming the pregnancy isn't terminated by choice. These stereotypes are depicting reality less and less. One result of them is that increasingly women who are struggling to achieve or sustain pregnancy feel there's something fundamentally wrong with them on a deep human level, quite apart from their accidental physiological misfortunes.

Our society seems to be in denial of the fact that so many women are struggling to have babies. This may be due in part to a burden of unrealistic expectations being placed on women, who are supposed to balance career demands (often ones that would severely test any man) with the biological, psychological, and time-management demands of motherhood as well. As women postpone motherhood in favor of first launching a career, more are becoming pregnant at ages exposing the pregnancy to high risk. There needs to be more public conversation about this to help dispel the feelings of personal abnormality and inadequacy which weigh so heavily on many women who experience age-related pregnancy complications. Talking more openly about it will also help inform more women in this position about how much can be done to help them. To many, this discovery comes as an enormous emotional and intellectual liberation from the oppressive "inevitable cycle of miscarriage" culture in which misinformation traps so many aspiring mothers (and fathers). This culture preys on the minds of women who suffer miscarriage. As if pregnancy loss were not traumatic enough they're made to endure a guilty sense of having failed womanhood itself. These issues have to be faced in order to get the most out of the womb knowledge presented in this book.

Chapter 3

∽

YOU'RE NOT ALONE!

One of the cultural problems that make high-risk pregnancy an even worse experience for women than it need be is the dangerous idea that, to be a modern woman, you have to be supremely self-sufficient.

A healthy sense of individuality is good, but it's also healthy to know that, male or female, you belong to something that transcends individuality. My clinical experience has led me to believe that this awareness is essential to a successful pregnancy experience. The expectant mother must accept that her pregnancy confronts the limits of her selfhood.

How so? First, pregnancy (at least at this point in history) means someone else had a role in transforming your body. Second, pregnancy requires you to share your body with another being: the baby emerging within you. Third, perhaps more than any other experience, pregnancy demonstrates that no human life is isolated. Every pregnant mother's story is part of the story of all the women who've ever been pregnant over the millennia. You're part of a great choir to which millions of women have contributed their unique voices. Fourth, your pregnancy experience is entitled to inherit and benefit from the knowledge that we've accumulated from all that vast sisterhood. You are not alone. It will help you enormously to deal with pregnancy challenges if you can conquer the feeling of aloneness that these problems can foster. By drawing on our society's accumulated pregnancy knowledge to achieve an optimal cooperation with the ancient wisdom of the body, 21st-century women have formidable advantages over earlier mothers. Pregnancy was once so hazardous it's hard to read about childbearing experiences of even a few decades ago, let alone centuries or millennia, without shuddering. There used to be good reason for the old proverb, "A pregnant woman has one foot in her grave." A study of ancient mummies in South America found that 14% of the women between 12 and 45 died of childbirth problems. [9] Scientific advances make today's women much better off.

This doesn't mean the risk has gone out of having a baby. On the contrary, science has enlarged our understanding of the extent and nature of the risks. We now know that any one of a vast number of factors can change your pregnancy at any moment. The line between a healthy pregnancy and a problematical one is very fine. And yet, at no time in history have pregnant women been armed with more knowledge than is available to them today. The sense of hopelessness that comes to so many women facing pregnancy complication arises too often without any realization of this fact. If you are struggling with any of the types of pregnancy complication that I describe in these pages, and if you are willing to act on the information I offer, you may have a much more realistic reason than you may think to hope for a healthy, full-term baby, despite your history or fear of pregnancy problems, including even multiple miscarriages.

Most importantly: you're not alone. There's a mass of knowledge to help you, and despite the barriers, you can find people willing to help put this knowledge to work on your behalf.

The psychological and cultural attitudes to pregnancy that I've mentioned now lead me back to talk about a common mistake in thinking about pregnancy. (I indicated it briefly earlier.) This error, which is relevant to just about everything in this book, is that pregnancy is somehow a fragmented phenomenon consisting of events that happen separately and at different stages, without having much to do with one another. Contrary to this mistaken idea, pregnancy is in fact a unified phenomenon which can be properly understood only in its integrated totality. A good way to explain this is to draw to your attention that I've spoken of the challenge of sustaining a pregnancy through to a successful outcome, as distinct from the obviously related but nonetheless different challenge of becoming pregnant. Now, this distinction between becoming pregnant and sustaining your pregnancy is part of the vocabulary of distinctions that sciences use to arrange information into different compartments. This analytical practice is not just helpful but essential to scholars and scientists when they have to organize huge amounts of information into clear patterns that our minds can manage. But what many learned people often forget is that the diagrams and patterns we invent to help us organize information are abstractions that we artificially impose on nature. Nature itself doesn't organize itself into neat compartments. It's untidy and often unwilling to stay within the artificial lines that human minds find it so useful to draw between different objects and processes. The human body is one of the best examples of this love that nature apparently has for connecting things which, to the simplifying human eye, don't seem to have anything to do with each other.

The history of science, especially medical science, has largely been a story of discovery of how different phenomena are connected with each other in previously unsuspected ways. We're constantly learning more about how the various parts of the human body aren't distinct from each other, as when we draw them in a textbook, but in fact interact with each other. At the same time, we're endlessly discovering formerly unknown connections between our bodies and our environments, including the technologies we use, the air we breathe, our food, our medicines, the substances out of which we manufacture things, and the trappings of the lifestyles we choose or which circumstances impose on us. This interconnectedness is one of the most remarkable aspects of the ecologies of which we are all part. There is a moving beauty of this great scheme of links joining all the processes of living and inanimate nature into a vast unity, in which circles within circles of interwoven phenomena underlie the loveliness of scientific truth. And it's all made all the more enchanting by the inevitability that no sooner do we become satisfied that we know all there is to know about something, than a startling new perspective shifts into view, shattering our comfortable habits of seeing and thinking. These features of science, life and human understanding are beautifully illustrated by pregnancy. Gaining insight into the extraordinary unity of all aspects of pregnancy is the key to pregnancy wisdom, and to your ability to navigate successfully through the dangers that threaten to interrupt pregnancy before a healthy birth can occur.

Earlier I spoke of the developmental stages through which every pregnancy passes, or strives to pass, as reflecting a unity of both space and time. By unity of space, I mean that the health of your pregnancy is determined not just by what happens in the womb but also by what takes place throughout the rest of your body as it responds to your pregnancy. By unity of time, I mean that what happens in the very earliest stages of your pregnancy shapes events that occur at every subsequent stage, down to the moment the pregnancy ends. This doesn't at all mean that what happens at the outset of your pregnancy determines its final outcome like an iron law. But regardless of whether you experience a miscarriage or deliver a fine and fully healthy baby, or a baby who is alive but afflicted by abnormally low weight or inadequate development in some other way, the outcome will have been influenced to at least some degree by preceding events going back, possibly, to the time you conceived, or shortly after conception, or even before conception, as well as by things that you did at various stages throughout the entire duration of the pregnancy, or by actions which you or your doctor should have taken during those months but, for whatever reason, did not. Certainly, from the moment you become pregnant, everything matters. There is no such thing as being concerned too early about pregnancy health.

I've noticed that most women seem to have an intuitive understanding that all the events of pregnancy form a unified totality, yet medical custom runs counter to this understanding because of the compartmentalizing I've described. Even though scientific knowledge advances by discovering connections, there's apparently a belief that dividing things into compartments is somehow inherently scientific. In my opinion this influences doctors considerably, and this problematic influence is exacerbated by the fact that dealing with things in their parts rather than as a whole justifies a convenient focus on just one aspect of a pregnancy at a time, an approach that doesn't always meet the pregnancy's needs. For these reasons I agree with British sociologist Professor Ann Oakley's remark that the character of modern medicine is "largely unscientific."

Now, because pregnancy isn't a series of isolated events but a complex process in which every stage is important, I'm going to talk in coming pages about every part of this process. But my focus here isn't on the difficulties that some women experience in becoming pregnant. I'm focusing rather on staying "in business" once you achieve pregnancy: that is, on avoiding miscarriage and other pregnancy disasters. Which leads me to one of the most heart-rending cries of women who experience miscarriage, especially recurring miscarriage. This cry always takes the form of an angry, frustrated, desperate question:

Why is this happening?

Chapter 4

CAREER FIRST ... OR BABIES FIRST?

If you haven't been in a pregnancy situation that drove you to ask this question, I'm happy for you. But I want you *to never* have to ask it.

I've talked a bit about the thinking that went into the writing of this book, including its choice of title, The Working Womb. This title reflects the natural desire, indeed the reasonable expectation, that your womb should work as it's supposed to. To act on this desire, you need to know how a healthy womb works. But the title has another nuance, one that I've already introduced and must now discuss further. In today's world, a womb is increasingly likely to belong to a woman who has a paying job outside the home. This is the age of the working woman, and as I've already indicated, this inevitably has implications for what happens in the womb.

In generations past, having and raising babies dominated most women's lives, but today, more and more women pursue a career before fulfilling all their pregnancy aspirations, or even before having a first baby. It's one of the most significant developments of our age that women are deciding to become pregnant later and later in life.[10] I commonly treat women who in previous generations would have been considered well past child-bearing. This phenomenon of increasingly later motherhood underlies many of the pregnancy complications I treat, since advancing years put a mother at greater risk of various types of complication.

Pregnancy disorders shouldn't be disproportionately blamed on this phenomenon, though. Many recurring pregnancy problems have origins in earlier pregnancies when the mother was much younger. Those earlier pregnancies can hold the seeds of problems which in time grow prominent enough to jeopardize the patient's later child-bearing. The blindness of many doctors to the connections between pregnancies is part of the inattentiveness to the sense of process I've mentioned. It's not only the various phases of each pregnancy that must be taken into account in a unified context but also the links between all the mother's different pregnancies.

It's significant to speak of different pregnancies because, while every pregnancy forms part of the totality of the mother's physiological experience, each pregnancy isn't just different numerically, in that it's first, second or third, but unique in terms of what happens in the womb during that particular pregnancy, including its own unique medical risk factors. The effects of these risks aren't limited to the single pregnancy in which they occur but can have ripple effects through the mother's life, affecting all of her health, including her later attempts to have a baby. Many a woman comes to me in tears after a doctor described her miscarriage or other pregnancy disorder as a one-time accident of mysterious cause, then the explanation is found after we examine her earlier pregnancy experiences.

The emergence of the working mother, or more accurately the woman who combines a career with motherhood aspirations continuing into mid-life, has now made it essential to look at all earlier pregnancies, successful or unsuccessful, when diagnosing pregnancy complications. For the same reasons of physiological continuity, a young pregnant woman of apparently unproblematic child-bearing age should realize that her seemingly straightforward, healthy pregnancy may contain seeds of disorders which can develop with time, threatening later pregnancies. Thus, for women to exercise their freedom of choice to pace their pregnancies consistently with career interests, doctors must grow accustomed to viewing all of a woman's pregnancy experience as a continuous child-bearing process. By the same token, the more flexibly a career woman wishes to exercise her pregnancy, the more she needs to know about her risks.

Of course, a pregnancy problem may originate not in an earlier pregnancy but in something that happened in the early stages of the very pregnancy that is now threatened. When this happens it's vital to detect the first sign of trouble when it occurs, rather than later. This means monitoring the pregnancy from the outset. Understanding why a pregnancy goes wrong is somewhat like investigating a crime. The sooner the detective gets to the scene to study the evidence while it's still fresh, the better; the later the detective arrives on the spot, the harder it is because the passage of time has obscured crucial evidence. It's my impression, unfortunately, that many doctors don't enjoy diagnostic detective work, preferring to confine themselves to looking up the more obvious and conventional diagnoses that are encouraged by medical habit. Reluctant to probe more deeply when the facts don't fit these prepackaged diagnoses, they prefer to tell the patient there's no real explanation; it's just "something that happens in nature." This kind of non-answer inflicts monstrous torment on a mother who's struggling to sustain a pregnancy and has been through hell because she feels in her deepest being that there must be an explanation as to why her womb doesn't seem to be working as it should.

My own experience is that when the womb appears to go on strike a reason can usually be found, and in a surprising number of cases it can be persuaded to go back to work. The problem most often turns out to involve your placenta. This is especially so for older women, but also for women with any medical issue that could lead to pregnancy complications. A working womb is one with a healthy placenta.

~

I spoke earlier of the need to learn to negotiate with your womb. In matters of placenta health, the womb is remarkably amenable to negotiation. The willingness of your body to cooperate with you is, in fact, demonstrated by the increasingly later age at which women are having healthy babies in the face of medical obstacles that would have made successful pregnancies impossible in earlier times. This is happening because much clinical experience has shown that proper respect for the placenta can have happy results, even in the face of apparently great obstacles. And this brings me to complete my choice of the title of this book.

In discussing pregnancy complications it's appropriate for the word "work" to be emphasized because ... well, having a baby in the face of any serious complication is a lot of work. For doctors, for the father, for other supportive family members, and most of all, of course, for the mother. I sometimes think because the issue of unwanted pregnancies is so hugely important, the public attention it receives unfortunately overshadows the ordeals of women who want a baby but struggle to sustain a pregnancy. Even as you read this, thousands of would-be parents are sick to the depths of their hearts because of how hard they're having to work at the seemingly natural act of keeping a pregnancy going. For these women there's an even greater than usual significance in calling the final phase of child-bearing "labor." In fact, my clinical experiences have taught me that applying this word only to the events immediately before birth is a misnomer. For many expectant parents, the entire pregnancy is filled with nail-biting stress. For months on end and sometimes (after serial miscarriages) even for years, the lives of these embattled couples are dominated by incessant work to pursue their dream to have a baby. The narratives of these couples are protracted dramas of physically and spiritually exhausting labor, requiring almost superhuman patience, persistence and determination. They battle feelings of inadequacy, personal failure, frustration and isolation in the face of widespread ignorance about what this kind of struggle costs aspiring mothers and fathers, emotionally and in many other respects. They're like soldiers fighting a war on behalf of life itself.

A high-risk pregnancy is a tremendous test for both parents as to what they want out of life and how much they want a baby. It tests the mother's relationship with her body. (All of us tend to take our bodies for granted.) It can test your friendships since even initially stalwart friends can tire of the support needed by a mother experiencing a complicated pregnancy. It can test one's finances, especially when health insurers balk at paying for the treatment a mother thinks is best for her. It can severely test your relationships with doctors, especially when you end up going for help from one doctor to another and still another. Worst of all is that it can even test your belief that you're fit to be a mother.

So when I speak of work in connection with the womb I refer not only to working women, and to your need to know how the womb itself works, but also to the grueling work that awaits many couples if they are serious about wanting a baby. However, this warning is balanced by the fact that your womb and your placenta will support your pregnancy mission with astounding resources if you work with them.

Chapter 5

THE MAKING OF A PLACENTA

If your body were an art gallery, we'd think of it as being filled with masterpieces, with your placenta as a supreme marvel.

Once you become pregnant, your placenta starts to grow on the inner lining of your uterus. Think of a bowl, eight or nine inches in diameter and two inches deep. Now picture yourself digging up a small plant, washing out the dirt from its roots, and tucking it snugly into the bowl. Pat it down so the roots fill the bowl neatly. Now seal the bowl securely with plastic wrap. That's pretty much what your placenta looks like. On one side it's joined to your body's complex system of veins and arteries; the other side will link to your fetus's circulatory system. This arrangement will allow your unborn baby to share the nutrients and oxygen needed to grow and be born.[11, 12]

If you stay with the image of the placenta as a plant in a bowl, the plant's roots will represent small finger-like projections called villi that will contain the fetal blood vessels. The entire bowl will sit in a place with a science-fiction-sounding name: intervillous space. Before your placenta comes on the scene, this area belongs to a group of arteries connected to your uterus. These are spiral, i.e. coiled like mattress springs. During your pregnancy they'll uncoil as needed, expanding to match your placenta's growth. They connect to your uterus's inner lining, the endometrium. The placenta itself is formed as the blood vessels and glands in the endometrium multiply, grow and fuse with each other. The fetus's blood vessels will remain closed in the intervillous space, but the mother's blood vessels will open up into the space, emptying into it nutrients for the fetal villi to absorb.

But picturing all this isn't enough. You need to understand how the placenta comes to be.

~

Pregnancy begins with conception, when the father's sperm meets the mother's egg somewhere in the fallopian tube. Once the sperm enters the egg, its nucleus fuses with the egg's nucleus, becoming one. Each nucleus is a mass of genetic material containing all the instructions necessary to create a new person. These instructions are bundled into packages of information, like chemical versions of computer code. The packages are called chromosomes. To make a genetically normal human being you need 46 of them. The nucleus of a healthy sperm and the nucleus of a healthy egg each contain 23, so when sperm and egg come together as they should, they form a new nucleus containing the desired number of chromosomes. At this point, the process begins to resemble a formal dance because the 46 chromosomes don't come together in just any old way but arrange themselves (again, assuming they behave as they should) neatly in 23 pairs.

If all goes well, the result is an early-stage embryo which will be equipped to develop into a new, unique human being. This early embryo doesn't look anything like a person. It's essentially a little ball with an appetite. Every mother knows a healthy baby seems to be entirely made up of appetite, and this tendency is set right at the very outset. The moment it's formed, this microscopic ball inside you immediately needs to be fed. It absorbs food directly from the juices swirling around in your fallopian tube. A normal woman has two such tubes, one leading from each of your two ovaries. (When your ovaries produce eggs, the eggs travel to the uterus via the fallopian tubes. These were first described in the 1500s by an Italian physician, Gabriele Falloppio, to whom they looked like a musical instrument called a tuba; in his time this was not the same instrument that we call a tuba today, but was longer and more pipe-like.)

Once the early embryo takes shape, it doesn't sit still. Tiny hair-like structures called cilia, projecting from the fallopian tube's lining, stir up waves of motion that propel the early embryo to the uterine cavity, the space in the uterus that will become the embryo's home. The early embryo continues to develop while all this goes on, and although its development goes through various stages with different technical names. For convenience, I won't differentiate further among them and will just speak of "the embryo" from now on.

The embryo's journey to the uterine cavity usually lasts three to four days after ovulation. Once inside the uterine cavity, it will settle somewhere on the uterus's inner lining (endometrium). The surface of the endometrium is huge in relation to the tiny embryo, but not every spot is equally good for settlement. The embryo must implant itself where it's most likely to be successful.

As real estate brokers say, it's all about location. Compelling evidence indicates that powerful forces in your body work together to help your embryo find the best possible location. These forces start coming into play even before the embryo is formed. We know that a select area of the endometrium will start enlarging its blood vessels in preparation before ovulation! New vessels will also be created to provide plenty of nutrients and this area of the endometrium thickens, developing a rougher, velcro-like surface.[13-16]

Amazingly, the endometrium communicates with the embryo in advance of its arrival. It sends out special molecules (a molecule being a package of atoms arranged in a unique way). Research suggests that the endometrium's new "velcro" surface releases substances which boost this communication process, helping the embryo find its way to the optimal location, or "hot spot," where it will implant itself. All this happens in a climate of utmost urgency and suspense because if the embryo's journey to its designated hot spot takes too long, implantation will fail. Conditions remain right for the endometrium to welcome the embryo for only six to eight days at a time. This relatively tight window of opportunity explains why, during her fertile years, a woman has only a 15% to 25% chance of pregnancy in a monthly cycle.[13, 17, 18]

As the moment of implantation draws near, the embryo starts changing. It grows its own velcro-like projections to help anchor itself to the endometrium. This is a most perilous phase. Almost half of all embryos fail at this point. If the attachment doesn't work, this particular pregnancy will be over. On the other hand, attachment can succeed … but on a spot other than the optimal one. This could result in a pregnancy impaired by inadequate placenta development.

Another problem that occurs all too frequently is the development of twin embryos. The place on your endometrium that your body's processes identify for optimal implantation can be occupied and used for full growth by only a single embryo. If twin embryos arrive, one of them is left with little space for attachment in the vicinity of that desirable location. You could call this the earliest manifestation of sibling rivalry. The disadvantaged embryo can still implant itself, but, like Cinderella, it's going to be relegated to second-class status while the favored embryo receives the lion's share of resources. The Cinderella embryo's placenta won't develop properly. The results of this can range from discordant twin growth (significant difference in the weight or size of the twins) to premature birth and even the death of the unlucky fetus.

But let's focus for now just on the embryo that attaches successfully, so you'll understand what proper placenta growth and embryo development entail. Once it's successfully implanted, the embryo does what any new homeowner does: it starts putting its own personal stamp on its property. First, it produces chemicals that break down the top layer of the endometrium's lining. Then it projects some of its own cells, like feelers, down under the surface of the endometrium to link up with some of those spiral arteries I described earlier. These deep-burrowing feelers are the embryo's underground workmen. Like carpenters and plumbers, they go about transforming that section of the endometrium, altering not only the tissues directly under the successfully attached embryo but also the surrounding area below the endometrium's surface. Fanning out as they tunnel, wherever they find good blood vessels, they connect them to the embryo's network.

And now we encounter a most interesting phenomenon. Just as with any neighborhood, the endometrium isn't without its sense of exclusivity. It doesn't welcome just anyone. It has its prejudices. Bias against foreigners is found not only in this region but throughout every healthy human body, both male and female. The guardian of this prejudice is the body's immune system, which protects us against microorganisms capable of harming us. As I explained when I talked about Mary, when an invader like a virus or germ breaks into our body, the immune system sounds the alarm and sends armies of NK (natural killer) cells to attack and destroy the foreigner.[19]

But what about the embryo? Isn't it also a foreigner, in a sense? The answer is both Yes and No. Remember, half of the embryo's genes come from its mother. The immune system recognizes them. But the other half of the embryo's genetic material is from the father, and in principle it qualifies the embryo as a foreigner as far as the immune system is concerned. Despite this, the NK cells don't (in normal circumstances) attack the embryo. The reason for this is complicated enough to fill another book, but the short explanation is that special molecules called antibodies cover the foreign parts of the embryo and chemically disguise it as a familiar part of the mother's body. These molecules are called blocking antibodies. Due to them, the embryo can develop unmolested.

What I've described happens in normal circumstances, but abnormalities can occur at this stage of the pregnancy. Sometimes the mother's body has an auto-immune disorder, in which her immune system is confused and the NK cells attack the placenta tissues (as happened to Mary) despite the disguising work of the blocking antibodies. This activity is a cause of recurrent miscarriages.

Before we get further into abnormalities, let's return to the embryo that's securely implanted in the optimal part of your endometrium, its feelers becoming longer and penetrating more deeply into the subsurface endometrial tissue. Around three and a half to four weeks from the first day of the mother's last menstrual period, the embryo's first feelers will reach their first spiral artery, and it's now that the heavy work begins. [20-22]

First, the feelers destroy the outer wall of the spiral artery and break through to the artery's inner layer, which consists of muscle cells. Next, the feelers set about digesting these muscle cells, by giving off chemicals which break the artery muscle cells down into a form which the feelers absorb as foodstuff. As each spiral artery muscle cell is digested, the feelers don't leave an empty space in its place but replace each digested cell with substitute material, like a bricklayer who, during a renovation, removes bricks from an old wall and replaces them, one by one, with new bricks that are more to the homeowner's liking.[23, 24]

This has a very important result. The flow of blood through an artery is controlled by tightening or relaxing the muscle cells that the embryo's feelers have now started to replace. When the muscle cells tighten, less blood is supplied to the surrounding body parts. When the muscle cells relax, more blood is supplied. Usually, this contraction-relaxation rhythm is automatic, being regulated involuntarily by your nervous system. During pregnancy, however, the embryo uses the muscle-cell digestion process that I've just described to hijack control of the spiral arteries, like a hacker taking over a computer system.

By replacing the muscle fibers of blood vessel walls with cells that it controls, the embryo can meet its increasing food and oxygen demands by dilating the vessels as needed. To appreciate the importance of this, you need to understand what the flow of blood to your uterus means to your fetus. In a non-pregnant state, your uterus is not larger than a fist. It receives blood via two main uterine arteries. In a non-pregnant woman, about 50 milliliters of blood (say, three or four tablespoons) are delivered to the uterus every minute via both of these two main arteries. This blood is circulated by branches that lead off from the arteries. Each main artery splits into two branches, one going down and the other up. The downward one supplies the cervix (the part of the uterus that meets the vagina); the upward-turning one supplies the body of the uterus itself.

I described the placenta earlier as a bowl representing an open area in the body called intervillous space. Well, after the embryo takes control of the spiral arteries, this space is flooded with the mother's blood. This nutrient- and oxygen-rich blood then bathes the finger-like projections (villi) that contain blood vessels servicing the embryo. These vessels now freely absorb from the surrounding blood all the food and oxygen they need.

When the embryo has taken everything it can from a unit of blood, that "used-up" blood is absorbed into the mother's veins (which differ from arteries in that they don't deliver blood but take it away). The depleted blood is taken away and stocked up with a fresh supply of food and oxygen to bring back to the embryo. And the "used" blood that returns to the mother's veins doesn't go empty-handed; it carries with it the embryo's waste products, thus providing not just food and oxygen but also a garbage disposal service, the garbage consists of carbon dioxide gas and by-products of metabolism (the chemical processes whereby the embryo uses its food to grow).

The embryo's villi absorb food directly from the mother's blood through the villi walls and deposit waste into the mother's blood in the same way, so the villi walls must be just the right thickness. If the villi walls get too thick (or if the mother's blood is too thick), the embryo doesn't get enough food and oxygen. It then won't grow properly, and if this goes on too long it will die. If the problem is eased in time the embryo can survive, but it may be damaged beyond repair. A baby born from such a deprived pregnancy may, for example, have an increased risk of developing blood clots in later life. Everything in this process is very finely balanced. Conditions have to be just right to be optimal for the growth of the healthiest baby you can deliver. Because a healthy embryo's ability to command the blood supply is essential to placenta functioning (and to a successful pregnancy), the taking over of the spiral arteries is the very foundation of how the placenta comes to be.

As we've seen, there are two main uterine arteries, the right and the left. Each splits into an ascending and descending artery. The descending one becomes the cervical artery; the ascending one supplies the uterus and the placenta. The ascending one isn't straight, but folds and winds, much like the spiral arteries, and for the same reason: to be long enough to stretch and match the uterus's steady enlargement to fit the growing fetus. It also now grows branches, forming a kind of basket around the uterus. To visualize better how this system delivers oxygen and food to the embryo, let's take an imaginary trip. In 1966, a popular movie, Fantastic Voyage, revolved around the idea of a technology enabling people and things to be shrunk to a very tiny size. The story was that an important man went into a coma and a blood clot threatened to kill him, but it was too dangerous to operate, and of course the only way to save him was for a group of brave people to be shrunk and injected into this unfortunate man's body. Once inside him, they traveled through his bloodstream in a miniature submarine to destroy the clot with a laser beam.

Chapter 6

FETUS OR BABY?

If you were to approach the heart in a tiny submarine it would not be a quiet experience. You would hear the tremendous sound of the heart's beating. It seems only fitting that a relentlessly pounding masterpiece of muscles, nerves and electrochemical impulses should make itself known and felt within the body by a great noise. In our microscopic form, this noise drowns out our speech, as if in a mark of our respect for this majestic booming within your chest which, astonishingly, goes on and on without resting all the years of your life as your heart faithfully fulfills its duties as the central engine of your body.

The pervasive rhythm of sound and vibration that emanates from the heart is created by the orderly expansion and contraction of the muscles of this amazing organ. To complete the symphonic pattern there is, in the background of the beating, a constant waterfall music which is the rush of blood flowing through the heart chambers as the pumping drumbeats admit each unit of the bloodstream into its chambers and then expel it with a renewed blast of propulsion to send it on its return journey through your body. When the blood is thus propelled away from the heart, it will have a new shipment of oxygen to carry to its designated ports. In order to align our mental picture with biological fact, we must imagine that the portion of blood that we're riding into the heart has come straight from the lungs, where it's just taken on a fresh load of oxygen. The red corpuscles zooming along with us are now fully loaded with their precious cargo.

We enter the heart by passing into its left side, the entry zone for all blood, the heart's right side being kept busy with sending blood to the lungs to pick up fresh oxygen. Our submarine sails us into a thundering cavern called the left atrium. Architects use the term atrium to describe a type of space inside houses and other buildings, usually leading into other rooms. This sense of the word applies in the heart too, for the left atrium is a foyer for oxygenated blood coming from the lungs, and this newly resourced blood is immediately directed into another chamber, the left ventricle. The left ventricle's walls do the tremendous squeezing that rockets the oxygen-replenished blood back out of the heart and on its way around the body to deliver oxygen wherever it is needed.

In our microscopic submarine, getting from the left atrium into the left ventricle would be a violently turbulent ride because the gate between these two chambers consists of two flaps which keep opening and shutting automatically. Think of those revolving doors, or other kinds of doors which automatically open and close by themselves, in which children often play by hopping in and out before the doors can touch them. This is the kind of exact timing we'd need in order to get through the doorway between the two heart chambers before the flaps swat us. (This doorway is called the bicuspid valve, or the mitral valve, because it looks like a miter, a hat that bishops wear.)

Imagine, now, the valve flaps opening lightning-fast and the blood in the atrium (including our submarine) being turbo-boosted through. Inside the left ventricle, the blood is tumbled and spun in a cascade of colliding waves that are at once like a whirlpool, a waterfall and the rapids of a white-water river; all this upside-down tumult takes just a second or less before the decisively contracting walls of the left ventricle shoot out a jet of oxygenated blood on its assigned way around the body. Inside this geyser blast our submarine makes its pummeled way, and we find ourselves in another flooded tunnel: the ascending aorta.

The ascending aorta is part of your body's biggest artery, the aorta. The whole aorta is shaped somewhat like a candy cane, being a straight tube, except for a short curved section at the top, which is the ascending aorta. This ascending section leads out of the heart, and, when newly oxygenated blood is shot out of the heart into that short aortic tube, what happens is the opposite of the way a roller coaster works. In roller coaster rides, you go uphill slowly, and then at the top of the hill you go down like a bullet out of a gun, with the wind pressing you back against your seat so you lose your breath. But, in the ascending aorta, it is the upward journey that has great speed because the blood that travels upward has behind it all the force that the heart can muster, which is formidable. Then, once the top-of-the-hill curve has been passed and the downward trip has begun, the bloodstream puts on the brakes, and the blood goes down the descending aorta at a more relaxed pace.

This downward part of the aortic journey takes us through the chest and into the abdomen, past openings that branch off into the arteries delivering blood to your liver, intestines, kidneys and elsewhere; but these stops aren't important to us today. We must focus just on how replenished blood delivers oxygen and food to your uterus, your placenta and ultimately your embryo.

At the entrance to your pelvis, the aorta splits into two branches called the iliac arteries. One goes down the left side of your pelvis, the other down the right side. As each iliac artery descends further down the pelvis, it splits again into two branches called the external and internal iliac arteries. The internal iliac artery takes us into the uterine artery. This artery once again has branches leading off it, this time to the arcuate arteries. ("Arcuate" means they're shaped like a bow.) Eventually, this system of increasingly branched arteries ends in offshoots which lead off in various directions like the spokes of a bicycle wheel or rays from the sun; hence their name: radial arteries.

The radial arteries go through the myometrium, or middle layer of the wall of your uterus. The myometrium, containing a lot of muscle tissue, will enable your contractions when you give birth, so it needs to be assured of a good and constant supply of nutrients and oxygen. On either side of the myometrium, sandwich-like, is another layer of the uterine wall. The outer layer is the perimetrium and the inner layer is the endometrium, in which the embryo we've discussed has implanted itself.

We now have a mental picture of what blood is made of, what it does, and how it gets around. These images provide the framework for the scene I must describe next. We've seen how the descending aorta leads to the iliac arteries, one of which becomes the uterine artery, which in turn branches until it leads into the radial arteries. These penetrate the wall of your uterus until they reach the inner portion of the myometrium that borders the endometrium. Shortly before the radial arteries reach the endometrium, they branch into arteries which extend sideways to the base of the endometrium, hence their name: basilar arteries. A small portion of the ends of the radial arteries and the beginnings of the basilar arteries transforms into the helicine arteries. (Named for their helix-like shape.) Finally, the helicine arteries penetrate the endometrium and branch into an even more helical form, being coiled like a mattress-spring; these are the spiral arteries we met much earlier. This is the final branching of the uterine artery system.

Just as rivers pour their waters into a lake or sea, so the spiral arteries bear blood into the intervillous space, creating a lake of enriched blood. This space, you will recall, is the open area between and among the villi (finger-like projections) that sprout from the embryo. A constant supply of enriched blood flows from the spiral arteries and bathes this space, allowing food and oxygen to be absorbed from the blood into the villi to nourish your embryo through all the stages of fetal development. So if we conclude our imagined journey in the little submarine, we find ourselves having travelled through all these many arterial branches, passing into ever finer and more delicate branches, until we now come to one of the coils of the spiral arteries, where we go round and round until we reach the very tip of the spiral, where at last we are released into the lake of rich blood that will nourish the growing embryo. And as we emerge from our turbulent arterial ride we find that although the fluid around us is calmer now, the endometrium itself is the site of much activity. The implanted embryo is very busy.

But before we inspect what the embryo is up to, this is a good time to clear up an issue that is bound to arise sooner or later. I've talked about embryos and fetuses, but when does an embryo become a fetus? And when does a fetus become a baby?

Many terms are used to identify the variety of stages that exist in the process that follows conception. I explained earlier that because this isn't a medical textbook, I've chosen my use of medical terminology in general throughout this book. I think any mother should know, though, that physicians call the earliest stage of the embryo a zygote, and the next stage a morula (which sounds like the name of a drink), and the one after that a blastocyst. These names describe the development of the embryo over the first eight weeks. From the 9th week, doctors will refer to a fetus until birth, at which stage the fetus becomes a baby. But most people talk and think not in medical language but in the ordinary language of everyday life, and in this language I've found that mothers and fathers think of their unborn offspring as a baby from Day One. No one knits booties for an embryo. After a miscarriage, people mourn the loss of a baby, not a fetus.

The most important emotion that an expectant mother can have, in my opinion, is a feeling of identification with, and responsibility for, the new individual taking shape within her. For this feeling to be possible, she has to think of this developing individual as a person, although with the understanding that she's really thinking of the potential person rather than actual being growing inside her. In this book, as in my clinical practice, I sometimes refer to an embryo, sometimes to a fetus, and sometimes to a baby. It depends on the context. But even where I refer to an embryo or a fetus, it will always be with the idea that I'm talking ultimately about stages in the development of your baby, in the sense of the baby you hope to have. As for the words that a pregnant mother herself chooses to use to describe the unborn life within her at various stages of pregnancy, that's up to one person alone. The mother.

Having digressed to clear up these points of terminology, I now return with you to the surface of your endometrium, which has become a scene of great activity as a home takes fuller shape for the implanted embryo in its wondrous mission of transformation.

Chapter 7

THE MYTH OF THE TRIMESTER

You'll remember we saw how the embryo's feelers destroy the outer wall of each spiral artery and set about digesting the muscle cells behind the wall, replacing each digested cell with substitute material of its own, thereby gaining control of the spiral arteries. Because of this takeover, the embryo can now dilate the "hijacked" spiral arteries to suit its needs, like adjusting a faucet to control the flow of water. This lets it access food and oxygen in the replenished blood at a pace that meets its pace of development. The number of spiral arteries that will be taken over will be at least 80 and could reach 180 or so. This takeover process will particularly affect two aspects of your emerging placenta's health. First, the more arteries that are successfully taken over, the healthier the placenta will be. Second, the deeper the takeover goes, the more oxygen-rich, nutrient-laden blood will be made available to your embryo, your fetus and your baby.

The takeover campaign lasts for 24 to 26 weeks and unfolds in two phases. Phase One, which lasts between 12 and 14 weeks, determines which spiral arteries are to be remodeled and how many. Phase Two, lasting about a dozen weeks after the first phase is finished, consists of your embryo's efforts to extend its control of the hijacked spiral arteries as deeply as possible into the length of these arteries.

The takeover is extensive, dramatically changing each artery. Before you become pregnant, your spiral arteries are each about one-fifth of a millimeter wide (around eight thousandths of an inch). By the end of the takeover, each spiral artery has the capability to stretch itself to up to 10 times wider. This enormous increase in size means these arteries can deliver much more blood to the uterus, which, in part, is why a pregnant uterus receives some 20 times more blood than a non-pregnant one. That is, before you become pregnant, your uterus makes do with about 50 milliliters of fresh blood every minute, but during pregnancy this supply is boosted to around 1000 milliliters a minute. This enables your uterus to commandeer some 15% to 20% of all your blood during your pregnancy.

Earlier I described how enriched blood would flow through to the spiral arteries to be released into the intervillous space, enabling the embryonic (and then fetal) villi to draw on its oxygen and nutrients. But this enriched blood doesn't start to be released into the intervillous space until after 11 weeks into the pregnancy. So how is the embryo nourished until then? In the early weeks of your pregnancy, before your bloodstream begins bathing the intervillous space, your embryo is nourished by two temporary sources, the yolk sac and something called the allantois. The yolk sac is a closed membrane, essentially a little bag. (The word "sac" is French for "bag", and is used in biology to indicate a bag that's part of a living being.) The sac I'm talking about is attached to the embryo more or less like a backpack, except that a backpack is usually attached to its owner, whereas here it's the other way round because the owner (the embryo) is smaller than the backpack. The embryo and yolk sac evolve together, but the sac is visible by ultrasound about five weeks into the pregnancy while the embryo is big enough to register only five to seven days later.

What happens is that, soon after you become pregnant, a membrane called the gestational sac is formed in the middle of the uterus. When you start going for your ultrasound examinations, the gestational sac is the first thing that shows up on the screen, generally in the fifth week. The yolk sac, which takes shape inside the gestational sac, is the next thing that can be seen. After the gestational sac and yolk sac become visible, the embryo itself is the third sign of pregnancy that the ultrasound detects. It's vital for the yolk sac to form properly; if it doesn't, the pregnancy will probably be unsuccessful, given the sac's crucial role in feeding the young embryo. (It performs this duty by using the chemicals inside the gestational sac that formed both the embryo and the yolk sac.)

When I spoke earlier about your red and white blood cells, I didn't mention that while these are manufactured in the marrow of your bones, every person's first red cells are produced by the yolk sac that nourishes them as an embryo. These first cells reach the embryo via the allantois at about five weeks. (In the later part of the first trimester, the embryo's liver takes over the production of red cells.) The allantois, too, is a kind of bag. It emerges more or less at the same time as the yolk sac, but it's shaped differently: its name comes from a Greek word, allantoides, meaning "sausage," which is what it looks like. The allantois is laced with veins and arteries, which equip it to serve temporarily as the embryo's circulatory system, providing the same kind of waste removal and nutrient supply functions that you receive from your adult bloodstream.

By the end of the first week after conception, the takeover of the spiral arteries in the uterus has begun to link your embryo to your bloodstream, but because the early-stage embryo isn't yet equipped to handle a lot of oxygen, maternal blood doesn't start entering the intervillous space in significant quantities until week 12 of the pregnancy. It's very important that your blood doesn't seep into the intervillous space too early. To ensure that this doesn't happen, the embryo forms plugs in the spiral arteries it takes over. If these plugs don't do their job well enough, and, as a result, blood leaks into the intervillous space before the embryo is ready for it, the premature delivery of oxygen can damage the embryo. If the leakage is big enough, the result will be a miscarriage. All this shows just how crucial these early weeks are for the health of your womb, and thus for your pregnancy. (By the way, "uterus" and "womb" mean the same thing, although we use "womb" specifically when we want to refer to the uterus's role as a home for the embryo and then the fetus, and as the place where structures like the placenta are formed and do their work; the word "uterus" tends to be used when we talk about this part of your body outside the context of pregnancy.)

Let's pause here to recap on these happenings of the first weeks of pregnancy. The arterial tissues of your uterus's inner lining, the endometrium, have started to join with the tissues of the embryo's projections, the villi. This two-way intermingling of the cells of the finger-like villi and the cells of the endometrium begins "weaving" a mesh of tissues that will eventually become the placenta. When this woven mass of tissues reaches its full size, surrounding your intervillous space and completely covering your original tissues, it's then your placenta, ready to do its essential work in seeing your pregnancy through to the day your baby is born.[12, 25, 26]

When it reaches this stage of full development, your placenta will probably be up to an inch (or a little less) thick in places. It will be linked to your fetus by a rope-like structure called the umbilical cord. This cord will be joined to the fetus at the place on the fetus which will in due course become your baby's navel. (The medical name for a navel is umbilicus.) The umbilical cord will grow up to two feet long. It's the growth of the placenta itself, though, that counts most. Studies show that the placenta's size in the twelfth week of pregnancy reflects the size of the baby at birth. The bigger (or smaller) your placenta is by week 12, the bigger (or smaller) your newborn baby will probably be. Here's a thought that's worth thinking about very carefully: if by the twelfth week your placenta is smaller than is desired for the best possible size and health of your baby at birth, it's too late to do anything about it.[27-29] Your doctor can't at this point make your placenta bigger if it's on the skinny side. The "missing" portion of an inadequately fleshy placenta just cannot be replaced. Once your placenta reaches the size it's going to be, it's final. It's then a matter of time before your unborn baby is affected by the reduced placenta size. I tell you this not to scare you but to give you knowledge you can use. I assume this book will be read by women who either want to become pregnant or who have just become pregnant. If you fall into either category, the good news is that you have time to benefit from what you learn from these pages. Which brings me to a major item of information that contradicts one of the most common beliefs about pregnancy. This is the fact that the "trimester" concept of pregnancy is a myth, at least in the form in which I've encountered it.

The idea that a pregnancy falls into three parts, or trimesters, is so deeply and anciently rooted in our culture that I'm fully aware of the professional risk I'm taking by exposing it as a myth. Among obstetricians, midwives, doulas and women everywhere, it's widely treated as a basic fact that nature has ordained pregnancies to unfold in three stages. This myth is perpetuated by the powerful forces of tradition and custom associated with the psychological appeal of the idea that it makes sense for important things to have a beginning, a middle and an end. In his study *The Number Three, Mysterious, Mystic, Magic*, scholar Emory B Lease notes that the ancient Greek philosopher Aristotle believed that the triad, or group of any three things, "is the number of the complete whole, inasmuch as it contains a beginning, a middle, and an end." Lease adds that "from time to time in the history of the world various numbers, chiefly those from 1 to 12, have been regarded as possessing a mystical significance, but there can be no doubt that in the extent, variety, and frequency of its use, the number 3 far surpasses all the rest... the study of the symbolic 3 takes us back to a remote antiquity, into the realms of mythology, religion, mathematics, philosophy, and magic – in fact, into almost every province of knowledge, to many and diverse lands, to people civilized and uncivilized, and to nations both ancient and modern."

It not only seems convenient or pleasing for us to divide things into threes, but there appears to be a kind of compulsion to do so, whether or not the thing that we're dividing into three parts has any physical or other factual basis for threefold division. If you look at an empty area of the sky or other space and decide to see it in three parts even though it's clearly an undifferentiated, continuous whole, who's to say you shouldn't? When we come to processes that develop over time, the naturalness of dividing the events into three can be even more plausible. The fact that in the theater, many plays have three acts may reflect such an underlying perception, perhaps connected to the idea of three seasons of human life: childhood, adulthood and old age, and to the notion that every process must start at some point and finish at some point, with everything else falling into a third section between the two.

The use of the word "trimester" to mean any three-month period (not necessarily in pregnancy) comes from the French trimestre, which in turn is derived from the Latin words tri (three) and mensis (month), while the use of the word to mean one of the three stages of a pregnancy seems to date back to at least the early 20th century. The trimester concept was given an important legal significance in connection with Roe vs Wade, the 1973 case in the Supreme Court of the United States where the court decided a woman has a Constitutional right to choose to have an abortion in the first two trimesters of pregnancy; in the third trimester, the court declared, government authorities could legally forbid an abortion. In another case, in the 1990s, the court dropped the Roe vs Wade trimester language and instead said that government could intervene at the stage when the fetus became "viable," whenever that might be. Whatever you think of these court rulings, the relevant thing for our discussion here is the court's recognition of the "trimester" approach to understanding pregnancy. The importance of this recognition didn't vanish when the revised wording was introduced. By giving the trimester concept this kind of legal recognition for many years, the highest court in the land further legitimized the concept, helping to entrench it further. Today the trimester concept is alive and well and is used every day to talk about care for pregnant mothers. Even when people recognize a need to change how we talk about pregnancy, they retain the three-trimester framework and expand on it rather than challenge it, so there are now references to "Trimester Zero" to refer to the period before pregnancy as well as to a fourth and even fifth "trimester" to denote events following birth. I applaud the recognition that pregnancy is too complex an experience to be limited to nine months. Doing so minimizes the importance of the parental behaviors and health factors that precede conception and yet greatly influence the pregnancy. It also underrates all those aspects of the baby's health which are rooted in womb events but don't end at birth, rather extending in impact throughout the newborn's growth all the way to adulthood. However, the new usages still feed on the trimester concept, which my clinical experience has convinced me is a myth. We must abandon the idea that pregnancy falls into three neat three-month compartments. It's ungrounded in physiological reality, imperils the health of both fetus and mother, and is a subjective notion which we've superimposed on pregnancy. It has no place in 21st-century medicine.

Pregnancy is a unity and a continuum containing the events that precede and influence conception, the events that follow birth, and the events and factors that carry over into the baby's future all the implications of what happened in the womb. It's also continuous during its nine-month process in the womb, in which the issues arising in each development stage are inextricably linked with the issues of the next stage. By minimizing these links, we create a false picture. To speak of separate stages of the pregnancy is a verbal convenience, helping us to manage information. In this sense, if we find it helps to think of trimesters, fine ... as long as we realize we're using a figure of speech. But words shape our habits of thought, and it's all too easy to allow them to shape our perception of the facts. The danger of "trimester" language is that it encourages us to see pregnancy as three neatly divided periods with tidy lines between them. It's a kind of Graduation Theory of the Womb, where your fetus first graduates from Trimester 1, then from Trimester 2, then achieves final graduation with birth. This suggests that once the fetus graduates from one trimester to another, all the needs of the trimester that's over have been successfully met and are now history, the way a student discards one academic grade's textbooks on being promoted to the next grade. This thinking can't be applied to pregnancy, least of all to placenta growth, which needs to have its earliest requirements taken into account from the beginning of the pregnancy and thereafter continuously, at every stage until you and your baby are home free. Your fetus does not automatically become safer the deeper you get into your pregnancy. The best way to explain this is for us to continue with the story of how the placenta develops.

Chapter 8

HOW YOUR BABY'S WEIGHT CAN DECEIVE YOU

On a very a fundamental level, your unborn baby (first as an embryo, then as a fetus) is in touch with exactly how your placenta is developing. Not consciously, of course. At the early stage of pregnancy I've been describing, the brain is still far from being formed, so there's no neurological basis for consciousness. But within the organization of cells that's developing into what will become your baby, genetic programming is at work, using chemical signals to obtain information about everything that is relevant to your pregnancy's success, with a special focus on how your placenta is coming along. And your developing baby isn't merely a passive receiver of this information. If all isn't going well with the placenta's formation, action is taken to correct whatever fault has been detected. But such correction comes at a price: as with the brain sparing I've described, the diversion of your womb's precious resources for remedial purposes upsets its finely-tuned budgeting, which can cause health problems even years later. So you have to do everything in your power to monitor the placenta's growth yourself. If there's any early growth restriction, and you identify its causes early enough to treat it, the placenta will catch up on its growth rate with minimal impact.

Here I'm talking about the first 24 weeks, when the invasion of the spiral arteries and other maternal tissues by your baby's cells is relentless, delicate and complex. Our computers are primitive by comparison. Indeed, long before the internet, iPhones or computers, the biological equivalent of super-sophisticated telecommunication had been going on for millennia in our bodies. One of the most astonishing examples of this is the signaling that happens during the embryo's assertion of itself into the uterus, when swarms of its signaling molecules bombard the maternal cells with the chemical "hacking" messages. These messages interfere with the programming of the mother's cells to allow the embryo to seize control of the spiral arteries, thereby defining the ultimate quality of the placenta and the subsequent health of the fetus.

When the remodeling of the spiral arteries is complete (24 to 26 weeks into the pregnancy), an important phase of placenta development is over.[30] From then on, the fetus will tend not to incorporate any more maternal tissues into the placenta's basic structure, although, if necessary, it can add some of its own cells to the placenta's mass to strengthen it.

By this time, around 24 weeks, the healthy placenta weighs close to a pound (just under half a kilogram), while the baby weighs roughly the same. By the end of the pregnancy the placenta may have gained up to half a pound, but the average baby will weigh seven and a half pounds (just under three and a half kilograms). So the ratio of fetal to placental weight at 24 weeks is about one to one, but at the end of the pregnancy it's somewhere between five and seven to one. Thus, the placenta reaches most of its size some 16 weeks before the baby reaches its maximum weight. This matters because the relationship between the weight of your placenta and the weight of your fetus governs the success of your pregnancy and the health of your baby. This profound fact is often disastrously overlooked when vital pregnancy management decisions are made. Which brings us to the Placental Syndrome.

A syndrome is a group of symptoms or medical conditions that tend to happen together or be associated with each other. The Placental Syndrome is so called because it involves complications related to placenta abnormality, including things most people don't think of as having to do with the placenta. As I've explained, my concern in this book is not with problems in conceiving but with problems in sustaining a pregnancy; however, appreciating the Placental Syndrome's importance is helped by knowing that it's relevant to conception difficulties as well. A woman with this syndrome may have experienced infertility and multiple IVF (in vitro fertilization) failures; she may have delivered a premature baby, or more than one; she may have had a baby whose growth was stunted; she may have experienced abruptio placentae (placenta detachment), or fetal demise, where the fetus dies in the womb after 20 weeks, or multiple miscarriages, or preeclampsia (high blood pressure during pregnancy), or neonatal death, where the baby is alive at birth but soon dies. All these conditions have this in common: a poorly developed placenta or a placenta that never forms properly at all.

But among the various medical experts who care for women experiencing such devastating pregnancy complications, a strange attitude prevails: they often tend to use the placenta as a scapegoat or convenient all-purpose excuse which can be invoked when a mother must be told that her pregnancy is doomed, or when, after the pregnancy has ended in disaster, she asks why she lost her baby. At such times it's very handy to be able to blame the placenta. After all, most people (even most doctors) know little about it, so how many mothers are in a position to challenge an expert who says the pregnancy failed because of this little-understood organ?

It's easy for a physician to tell a woman who has suffered a lost pregnancy that it's, well, "just the placenta." But it's the physician's job to read the placenta's calls for help in time. It angers me especially when these excuses for pregnancy failure are couched in religious language, as in "it was God's will for this pregnancy not to happen." Making the right diagnosis and applying the right treatment is a doctor's responsibility, not God's. This language is particularly reprehensible to me because it manipulatively plays to a stressed patient's emotions. Also, I've noticed that when a difficult pregnancy ends happily, some doctors will be happy to take the credit rather than attribute it to God. One of the most dreadful effects such cruel talk can have is to make a mother feel that God or life has judged her unworthy of motherhood. The psychological corrosiveness of such an experience can be shattering. I remember the case of a woman who had lost 12 babies and, every time, she was told there was nothing biologically wrong with her; each loss was either a freak accident or God's will.

In such cases, I tell the mother as quickly, forcibly and often as I can that she's certainly not responsible for events inside her that her doctor failed to diagnose in time, or for a misdiagnosis, or for a doctor's failure to prescribe effective treatment. These assurances are often poor comfort, and the best antidote I can offer, where circumstances permit it, is to assure her that, by following the right steps, she can still have a baby. So invincible is the impulse to motherhood that, armed with this information, even so traumatized a woman can generally come back from the brink of a total collapse of spirit, rebounding to answer the call that she knows will be made on her resources on behalf of the baby that is, after all, to come.

~

The placenta and the Placental Syndrome affect a much broader spectrum of women's health than pregnancy alone, and across a range of age that surprises many.[31, 32] The syndrome is associated with an increased death rate in women who have passed the age of menopause. This is because one of the most important areas of disorder in the placenta has to do with irregularities in the physiological mechanisms whereby a woman's body controls the clotting of blood. In recent years, especially with new methods to detect and measure clotting problems, it's become clear that women with clotting abnormalities are at increased risk for placenta-related pregnancy complications. Clotting problems can be devastating for placenta formation.[33-39] As long as the parents have healthy genes, a healthy placenta guarantees a healthy baby, but an abnormal placenta can result in a lost pregnancy, even if the baby is genetically perfect. Moreover, the same clotting problems that affect pregnancy also contribute to increased risk for cardiovascular disease after women experience menopause. More about this further on. What I want to emphasize now is that the placenta and the Placental Syndrome are connected not only with a mother's long-term health after pregnancy but also with the pregnancy's earliest moments. I see this in my long-term, follow-up work with patients, especially where multiple pregnancy efforts are involved. Here too, public understanding is distorted by false media stereotypes which foster the idea of childbirth as being exclusively about delivering a baby.

~

Back now to the story of the placenta's growth. By the 24th week, the placenta and fetus have reached roughly the same weight, but, halfway through the pregnancy, a healthy placenta will weigh more than the fetus … if early placenta growth has been healthy. If, in the first 24 weeks, growth is deficient for any reason, it will be hard for a doctor to detect this just by measuring the baby's weight with ultrasound. During this phase, the baby's needs will be satisfied even if the placenta is only half the size it should be. The baby's weight would in this case deceive you and your doctor. Because everyone's eyes are on the baby rather than the placenta, you and your doctor could remain dangerously unaware of the placenta problem. It's common in high-risk pregnancies for complications to arise from this "placenta blind spot" phenomenon, which is the background to many pregnancy disasters, since healthy fetal growth alone is not enough to achieve a successful pregnancy. The condition of the placenta is crucial. When I talked earlier about twin placentas, where one obtains the best spot on the endometrium, while the other is relegated to a less desirable one, I called the disadvantaged placenta a Cinderella. But if even a single placenta with a good endometrium spot is insufficiently monitored for healthy growth in the first 24 weeks, then it too is a Cinderella compared to the fetus, on which obstetricians commonly lavish most, if not all, of their attention. It's almost as if the placenta didn't matter during this critical period.

Obstetricians are my professional colleagues, and I'm not suggesting that this blind spot makes them bad doctors. They are simply following the prevailing habits of their profession. But because medical approaches can take decades to change, expectant mothers must be proactive to ensure they get the right care. You have more scope for action than you might think, not only regarding the limits imposed by prevailing medical custom but, for that matter, even in regard to the limits imposed by genes. In fact, understanding something about genetic limits will help you appreciate your power to influence your pregnancy outcome.

No doctor can make your baby healthier than its genes permit, but you can and must work informedly within the genetic limits. If you don't, you can certainly make your baby a lot unhealthier (even fatally so) than its genes allow. Working informedly within genetic limits means striving to make your placenta and baby as healthy as their genetic potential allows. This requires placenta progress to be monitored very early on. After week 24, your baby's growth rate will speed up enormously, and any previously undetected placenta problems will become obvious. You may now be told your placenta isn't right, and that consequently your baby isn't growing properly. If so, it will probably be only because the placenta has been ignored. You might also be told your own small body and inadequate weight are also causing problems; that the pregnancy must be observed very closely "from now on"; and, finally, that surgical delivery is needed to save the baby. The placenta will likely now be made the culprit, with your obstetrician in the role of a hero flying to your baby's aid. But your situation might well be expressly due to the prevailing attitudes of your obstetrician's profession. To avoid all this, you need to tell your doctor in good time that your placenta's early-phase growth is your top priority. Don't wait till disaster strikes. Tell your doctor early on you've learned that if the spiral artery remodeling in your womb has gone poorly, you face heightened risk of: (a) intrauterine growth restriction, i.e. impaired fetal growth due to food and/or oxygen deprivation; (b) losing your baby and becoming predisposed to later loss; (c) pre-eclampsia, involving high blood pressure and risk of eclampsia, involving maternal convulsions and the failure of the heart, lung, kidney, blood clotting and other systems (eclampsia can kill mother and baby and requires emergency delivery); and (d) cerebral palsy, where brain damage blocks control of various body areas. Failure to monitor early-phase placenta growth and take steps to correct growth imbalances in time is a sure road to trouble. The dangerous laxity about this all comes back to the Trimester Myth.

Completing the so-called first trimester with no warning signs isn't necessarily a cause to celebrate, as if you've passed a milestone entitling you to see the preceding three months as safely behind you. If untreated placenta problems have occurred during those preceding three months, they won't magically go away. This unfinished business will come back to haunt the pregnancy with a vengeance. The idea of hard-and-fast dividing lines between trimesters dangerously encourages a false sense of security, especially at the end of the first three months. Many doctors don't even see an expectant mother before week 12. Ironically, such "blind spot" misjudgment of the earliest weeks' importance is reinforced by their high mortality rate, which is shrugged off as just a fact of life. This circular reasoning fallaciously assumes that a problem's very existence somehow proves our powerlessness; it's just nature taking its course. In this philosophy, wisdom lies in doing nothing and waiting till the weak babies are weeded out so resources can be devoted to the tough ones who managed to make it through the first trimester without help. What a load of rubbish!

This is both clinically unfounded and shockingly callous.

This lazy thinking is related to the well-known phrase survival of the fittest, which suggests rationality and common sense require only the strong to survive, and "nature" (i.e. chance) decides who qualifies as strong. The phrase "survival of the fittest" draws on at least two ideas: (1) Darwin's Big Idea and (2) the idea of nature as a power transcending human influence (even though, paradoxically, this power also expresses itself through human action). These ideas directly influence the thinking behind conventional pregnancy management. Darwin's Big Idea refers to 19th-century scientist Charles Darwin, whose book *On the Origin of Species* gave us a convincing, evidence-based theory explaining how the traits of living things evolve over time by competing. The traits that prove most useful to survival are passed on in the bodies and behaviors of an organism's descendants, eventually creating life forms that differ so significantly from their ancestors that they're effectively a new being. However, the phrase "survival of the fittest," which summed up this Darwinian theory of evolution, was coined neither by Darwin nor any other scientist but by Herbert Spencer, a writer of popular books promoting competition (where the strongest and "best" contestants win) as the path to excellence. However, although the idea of competition is useful in many contexts, it's silly to elevate it into a supreme philosophy of life. Applying it to the ethics of clinical practice is misguided and certainly not scientific. For example, think of Marie Curie, who died in 1934. The Nobel Prize, given to the world's greatest scientists, was awarded to her twice, for her research in both physics and chemistry. (She pioneered the study of radioactivity.) Now, if she'd been born in a much earlier era, Marie Curie would likely have qualified as a weak member of society simply because she was a woman. Even if she'd managed to win some intellectual recognition she couldn't have done the scientific work we associate with her because it needed social support, which was unavailable in earlier times. Her deserved fame was made possible by a society which had the resources needed by specialized research. My point: Darwin's complicated theory is quite different from Spencer's simplistic slogan "survival of the fittest," and saying that temporarily weak things should be left to die is wrong and dangerous. This takes us to the idea of nature. To Spencer, competition was a dominant aspect of nature. In fact, though, cooperation is very natural. Humanity's natural ability to survive has crucially depended on amassing and using knowledge cooperatively, including medical knowledge. Despite the mistakes people have made throughout history, we all know that it's not in our deepest nature to shun cooperation, especially when it means abandoning those who can't protect themselves. If there's any place where this truth applies in its purest sense, it's in the care we owe the unborn.

It's sad that, in the 21st century, we should still be fighting this kind of battle on behalf of the unborn, but remember that many great changes in human behavior have changed painfully slowly, with inappropriate habits persisting long after overwhelming arguments pointed out their wrongness. Examples include slavery, the denial of voting rights to women, and smoking, which continues even today despite massive evidence about its grave dangers to health. When you consider how educated people can continue to ignore powerful evidence and arguments, it becomes easier to understand how the blind spot in placenta care, including the Trimester Myth, can persist despite clear clinical evidence that it endangers both mothers and unborn babies. My clinical observations have led me to conclude that in many cases complications and their effects, including miscarriages due to allegedly natural causes, result from this blind spot and insufficient attention to the placenta in that early phase of the pregnancy that's commonly called the first trimester. Such cases are to my mind not really miscarriages at all but unintended abortions. After 22 weeks, when the fetus starts becoming what doctors call "viable" (meaning it has some chance of surviving outside the womb), many doctors are more inclined to be prepared to watch the pregnancy closely. In my experience, there's no basis for this arbitrary timing. Why should a 10-week fetus be less valuable than a 22-week one? The prejudice against the early-stage fetus has no basis in medical fact and is entirely the result of custom. Can you, as a mother, do anything about all this? I believe you certainly can. Despite my severe criticism of the medical profession's conventional pregnancy management attitudes, most, if not all, pregnancy care physicians respect their patients and listen to what they say. But when you talk about the need to pay closer attention to the early stages of your pregnancy, it will help you to speak from a position of strength by showing some understanding of how pregnancy works. To that end, let's return to our discussion of the goings-on inside your pregnant body.

Chapter 9

YOUR WOMB'S AMAZING CAPACITY TO RECOVER

One of my chief aims is to overturn a common tendency in our culture to oversimplify the early stages of pregnancy, and to underestimate the complexity of the embryo itself, and then the even greater complexity of the fetus. Even in its very earliest phases, the embryo is far from being just a primitive blob. Though ranging in size from a pinhead to a grain of rice and then a garbanzo bean, the first forms of your unborn baby contain an immensity of genetically stored information representing eons of evolution. We've seen how this remarkable being establishes itself in a carefully selected place on the inner lining of your uterus, the endometrium, then sets about achieving control of your spiral artery system, creating a circulatory network which is woven into an increasingly dense mesh of blood vessel tissues, effectively growing an entirely new organ inside you: the placenta. We've also seen that your embryo's genetic information, derived from both parents, places limits on what your baby can become. But what

I haven't yet explained is the sense in which the embryo is also bigger than the sum of its inherited genes. To support its survival, evolution has given your embryo the astounding ability to change the way its genes work. This has enormous practical implications for the outcome of your pregnancy.

The idea of fixed genetic destiny is powerfully established in our culture. "It's in her genes" is another way of saying that someone's qualities are inescapably fixed, as if written in stone. I myself have told you no baby can become more than its genetic potential. But what does this really mean? It turns out that when it comes to answering this question, the human womb is like a clever lawyer who knows that in court you can argue only according to the law, but that the law can be interpreted in more than one way. And flexible interpretations come into play when the fetus encounters conditions which are so hostile that survival requires drastic action. Such action is called epigenetic imprinting. "Epi" is a Greek word with several meanings. The one that applies best here is "above": epigenetic imprinting means imposing something over the genetic instructions, or overriding them.

The fetus takes this emergency measure in response to a placental failure to provide sufficient food or oxygen. One of the reasons this is important to mothers is that if your fetus is driven to compensate for placenta failure in this way, it has to pay a price which may shape your baby's whole life after birth. Such a baby will weigh less at birth than its genes would otherwise have allowed, and it will in some ways always be less than it might have been. It might, e.g., have a poorly developed nervous system. This phenomenon of epigenetic imprinting is, in my experience, astoundingly poorly understood or even reported in the media. It's essential for you to gain insight into the kinds of placenta problems that can compel the fetus to override its genetic code. This information can be frightening, but it's balanced by what I have to tell you about your body's astounding ability to fix itself. (By the way, from now on, when I refer to trimesters, I use these terms not because I believe they have clinical validity but only for convenience. It would be tiresome to keep saying "so-called trimester." I've made my point that I don't believe in the trimester concept of pregnancy, so please bear this in mind as you read further.)

To understand the kind of placental threat that can trigger epigenetic imprinting, we must go back to the womb's intervillous space, into which, as I mentioned earlier, maternal blood doesn't normally flow until the 11th week. Such flow is present and easily detectable, though, in pregnancies which are heading for placental insufficiency. The premature flow of maternal blood into the intervillous space is associated with pregnancy loss, so its presence is a valuable warning signal.

We saw how, during the invasion and remodeling of the spiral arteries, the embryo forms plugs in these arteries to hold the mother's blood back until its appointed time for delivery into the intervillous space. If the plugs don't work well enough, blood leaks into the intervillous space before the embryo is ready for it, and this premature delivery of oxygen damages the chemically vulnerable embryo. You've probably heard of antioxidants, substances that protect your body from damage by certain oxygen-related chemical reactions. Antioxidants are present in fruits, vegetables, nuts and other foods. But your early-stage embryo hasn't yet developed antioxidant defenses, so if oxygen-rich maternal blood enters the intervillous space too early, the villi (those finger-like projections that are vital to just about everything that happens in your uterus during this period) will be damaged. This will weaken the development of the emerging placenta's ability to circulate the blood the fetus will need during the rest of the pregnancy. Such damage to the placenta's budding circulatory system can cause complications later in pregnancy, or even loss of the pregnancy in the first three months.

It's hard to overestimate the importance of those villi. Earlier, we saw that despite the mythical hard-and-fast borders that are commonly imagined as separating one trimester from another, the events of the first months of pregnancy don't contain their effects within those months but impact all fetal development that follows. Damage to the villi (or worse, their loss) in early pregnancy is a case in point. This can lead to significant loss of placenta surface in the last three months before birth, just when the fetus needs a full, healthy expanse of placenta surface to circulate lots of nutrients and oxygen. That's the worst possible time to find out that the placenta hasn't developed properly!

Now, your body is wonderfully resilient, with great capacity for self-repair, and some villi damage in early pregnancy can be corrected if the damage is caught early enough through timely examination, diagnosis and treatment. In most, if not all, cases where highly oxygenated blood prematurely enters the intervillous space, the unwanted oxidation will likely bring about thrombosis, causing blood clots which initially damage and eventually destroy the affected villi.[40] But, as soon as thrombotic conditions appear, they can be detected by ultrasound. Tests can then quickly pinpoint the cause of the premature blood seepage and the blood clots which are consequently forming. The two main causes of these conditions are chemical imbalances in the mother's own coagulation (blood clotting) system and problems in her body's regulation of its immune system.

Coagulation system problems can be very serious for both mother and baby. Both the embryo's successful implantation and the placenta's development depend on a healthy, delicate balance between clotting and anti-clotting mechanisms. If the blood clots too easily, it can't flow properly to deliver oxygen and food; if it doesn't clot enough or fast enough, there's bleeding, i.e. blood flows too readily and goes where it shouldn't. Both the mother's overall health and the health of the pregnancy therefore need just the right balance between the chemicals which cause clotting and those which restrain it. This balance must be stable and constant, with no erratic swings from one extreme to another.

Likewise, a well-functioning immune system is a prerequisite for healthy placenta development. The immune system's job to attack foreign presences is relevant to the fetal villi, which are, in a sense, foreign intruders, since they not only appear where they were previously unknown, but they also take over the spiral arteries in ways which look like a hostile invasion. The placenta too emerges in the uterus as a stranger, so it's unsurprising that even a normal immune system, let alone one which for any chemical reason has become oversensitive, should be alarmed. The result can be a dangerous immune-system response which disrupts crucial interactions between the developing placenta and the many spiral arteries whose job is to provide oxygen and nutrients to the uterine cavity. Like clotting issues, such immune system problems can be diagnosed with proper testing, but timely diagnosis and treatment depend entirely on whether the testing is done early enough as a result of thorough early-stage placenta monitoring. The timing is especially sensitive because some of these tests can't be done by the usual high-volume commercial laboratories but require special laboratory facilities. Once diagnosed, however, both clotting disorders and immune system disorders can be treated with medication.

If womb tissues are destroyed or even severely damaged by oxidation resulting from premature blood flow into the intervillous space, those tissues can't be restored. But the developing placenta is extraordinarily resilient and will respond with amazingly flexible and cooperative receptivity to any sign of help. The degree of its resilience is one of the most astonishing things I've learned in my work. It causes me great anguish to see how this potentially pregnancy-saving plasticity of the placenta seems to be either widely unknown or, even worse, sometimes known but simply ignored as irrelevant because of the myth that we can shrug off whatever happens in the early phase of pregnancy. In fact, sufficiently early detection and treatment of clotting and immune system disorders can not only stop the destruction of villi, it can also trigger the growth of new villi and fetal blood vessels. It's deplorable that this is so little known and understood by most physicians. Details about this regenerative capacity of the treatment-supported placenta are readily available but appear to be scarcely distributed among American pregnancy specialists. I myself have seen damaged placentas respond to treatment by recovering far beyond my expectations, and I can't sufficiently describe to you the awe evoked in me by the placenta's power to come back from disaster if only a helping hand is extended to it early enough. It's as if all humankind's anciently accumulated biological wisdom and will to survive has been concentrated in the placenta, just waiting for a medical hand of help to ignite an all-out effort to preserve the pregnancy. But, and I ask you to forgive what may be excessive repetition but I can't stress this too strongly, the placenta's recuperative capability doesn't cancel out the fact that once the placenta is damaged there's a limited window of opportunity to heal it. The earlier the diagnosis and initiation of treatment, the greater the scope for full placenta recovery. When the window of opportunity closes, the damage to the villi can be beyond repair, and you and your baby will be stuck with the consequences. Achieving timely repair requires you to ditch the false belief that the early period that's commonly called the first trimester doesn't matter as much as the rest of the pregnancy, if at all. If anything happens to prevent the process of spiral artery remodeling from being completed successfully, you and your baby face problems including recurrent pregnancy loss, pre-eclampsia, fetal growth retardation, cerebral palsy, fetal death, premature birth, premature rupture of membranes, and placenta separation (when the placenta becomes disconnected from the uterus).

To complicate things further, we still know little about the detailed workings of spiral artery remodeling. However, we can monitor the remodeling process closely with the latest ultrasound technology, which, unlike X-rays, doesn't expose the fetus to radiation.[28, 41-45] Long study has shown properly used ultrasound to be very safe, and, as a diagnostic tool, it's saved many babies. Thanks to it, we know that 73% of babies born with cerebral palsy have had thrombosis (abnormal blood clotting) in the placenta; also, that any form of placental thrombosis in the first three months is associated with a 75% chance of placenta-related complications, such as preterm birth, early pregnancy loss, cerebral palsy, placenta separation, severe growth retardation, late fetal death, stillborn babies, or other bad outcomes.

We've also learned that any bleeding during any stage during pregnancy is bad. It's widely believed that "spotting" (sporadic bleeding) during pregnancy is harmless. Not true! This is another myth in the cluster of misunderstandings about early pregnancy that explains why around a quarter of all pregnancies are lost. All bleeding in pregnancy is a warning of a problem that threatens a bad outcome … except if the mother has placenta previa (more about this later) in the first half of the pregnancy but is properly treated; in this specific case, some bleeding can be expected but won't necessarily signify a poor outcome. Bleeding from placenta previa in the second half of the pregnancy, however, can be lethal.

But now we must get back to the importance of timing and of your need to detect placenta problems soon enough to leave you enough opportunity to fix them. Let me tell you the story of the patient I'll call Miranda.

Chapter 10

MIRANDA'S CHOICE

This is a good case story to present here because it illustrates two of the matters I've discussed in recent pages: the importance of bleeding as a warning sign and the placenta's phenomenal resilience. Miranda was carrying twins. Her story started like that of many others but then developed, as has so often happened, into a unique series of events.

Miranda's first two pregnancies had miscarried. She was five weeks into her third when she sought the care of a specialist in maternal-fetal medicine at the suggestion of her obgyn (obstetrician-gynecologist), who'd discovered she had thrombophilia, in which inappropriate clotting happens. She was closely monitored and treated with the hormone progesterone, the blood thinner enoxaparin sodium, and baby aspirin. Things went well. After an uneventful full-term pregnancy, she had a healthy son. There was no reason to suspect what lay ahead in her next pregnancy, or how powerfully it would impact the pregnancies of many other women. Her case is a classic example of what can happen when a successfully diagnosed and treated pregnancy problem creates a false sense of security about the next pregnancy. Doctors often assume that because one baby's complications turned out well, it will be the same with the mother's next. With Miranda, as is frequently the case, this automatic optimism proved to be unjustified.

Following the success of her third pregnancy, she wanted to try again. For some two years, she struggled to conceive. She was sent to a reproductive immunologist (an expert on immune system problems affecting pregnancy), whose blood tests revealed that Miranda's immune system was excessively producing NK (natural killer) cells. This problem hadn't afflicted her previous pregnancies, but it was disturbingly relevant now. If she conceived, her body's abnormal alertness for anything that seemed foreign would likely identify her blastocyst (an early form of an embryo) as an invader. Her NK cells would attack it, preventing it from implanting itself in the uterus lining.

At the immunologist's advice, Miranda started a course of lipid (fat) emulsions administered by drip (intravenous infusions), which was known to suppress overactive NK cells. With further medical help, she became pregnant with twins, a boy and a girl. She was treated with anticoagulants for thrombophilia, a steroid (prednisone) for her immune issues, and lipid infusions for the increased NK activity. Then, around nine weeks, she began to bleed.

While the bleeding itself wasn't grave, it foreshadowed a crisis connected with severe placenta malfunction. Miranda had to get bed rest till the bleeding stopped and, for a time, things seemed to go well. At 12 weeks, a screening for Down Syndrome indicated her twins were at increased risk of developing this genetic condition, associated with intellectual and physical fetal impairments, but mercifully a further test showed this was a false reading.

Worse was to come. In keeping with accepted medical practice, Miranda was taken off prednisone between her 12th and 14th weeks and, shortly after, off lipids. Around three weeks later, one of the twins' growth had slowed disturbingly, and blood flow in its umbilical artery was severely irregular, with no diastolic flow (when the heart refills with blood). This was most ominous, and Miranda began to be even more closely monitored.

If one twin is normal, this helps to reveal abnormalities in the other, by comparison. At 17 weeks, I had to break the news that the girl twin's placenta was impaired. Blood flow wasn't good. A week later it was worse, with very little intermittent diastolic flow and no way to improve it. Each baby had its own placenta, but if one twin was delivered early, the other would have to be too, putting both twins at risk of serious damage, even death. It appeared the only way the boy twin could be allowed to reach full term and have a healthy delivery was by terminating his sister. This may seem to contradict my message that an early detection of problems can generate remedies, but it doesn't: in this case, termination was the standard-of-care recommendation at that time because there was no evidence then of any treatment that could change the outlook for this baby. If both babies had been allowed to continue, then even under the best circumstances one baby would likely have died (or been severely impaired) and the surviving one severely impaired, due to prematurity. In such circumstances, terminating one twin, as painful as it is, allows the other a chance to be born well.

At this point, possibly due to the stress and ischemia (insufficient blood supply) of one twin's placenta, Miranda's cervix, the neck-like lower part of the uterus leading down into the vagina, started shortening: it went from 42 millimeters to 26, a serious reduction. Both twins now faced death. Miranda was treated with indomethacin, the only anti-inflammatory tocolytic (an anti-contraction medicine used to prevent premature labor) known to lower the risk of premature birth. Indomethacin is the only medication that stops premature labor long enough to make a healthy difference. Because it can be taken only a few days a week, I prescribe it in conjunction with the second-best medication, nifedipine, which helps maintain the benefits of indomethacin.[46, 47] My clinic has demonstrated for the first time how indomethacin can be used as a tool to diagnose and treat patients with progressive cervical shortening. This approach improves cervical length significantly and reduces the need for cervical cerclage (stitching) to around 33% (without the use of indomethacin, 100% of patients with progressive cervical shortening require cerclage), significantly extending the time until delivery beyond 34 weeks in 95% of patients who were diagnosed with progressive cervix shortening between 12 and 28 weeks. Although these results have been published in the scientific literature, this treatment has not been integrated into the medical establishment's standard of care (currently conventional treatment approach). I believe most MFM specialists shy away from this treatment because using it safely and effectively requires exceptional knowledge of fetal cardiology and expertise in evaluating the fetal heart with ultrasound. If the treatment is used by a physician who lacks the necessary expertise, the baby could die. But the correct response to this challenge, in my view, is to require all MFM specialists to acquire the necessary knowledge. Until they do so, I believe, babies will in any case continue to die unnecessarily due to the fetal problems that this treatment regime can correct.

Under this treatment, Miranda's cervix returned to normal length and, although in most cases, mothers treated in this way don't need a cerclage, in her case, we decided that it was wise to give her this stitch. However, it looked like the problematic placenta was still unable to function adequately. In view of this, if we left things as they were, Miranda's own womb was likely to end her little girl's life support. In this event, her unborn son might also be lost in the physiological upheaval. This presented a dreadful choice: let one baby go, or try to keep it against the odds and thereby risk the life of its sibling.

Miranda couldn't accept that these were the only options. She felt there had to be another way. So began the worst time she'd ever known. She couldn't sleep, and although she didn't consider herself very religious, she started going to church, looking to the vocabulary of faith for the spiritual strength she needed to keep going. While her mind still groped for answers, deep down she knew with growing certainty that, no matter what, she wouldn't give up on her unborn daughter.

She decided to get a second medical opinion. To this I had no objection. When patients of mine feel that they need to consult another doctor with a different perspective, I encourage them to do so, not only because it is clinically ethical but because I understand that when one is confronted by appalling information, it's only natural and human to hope that perhaps different information will be available if only one knocks on a different door. And so, armed with all her case notes, Miranda went to a different high-risk pregnancy specialist, hoping he'd somehow be able to pluck a solution out of the air, as a stage magician appears to materialize a flower or a rabbit out of nowhere against all reason and evidence.

No such luck. The new doctor said the diminished blood flow

was even worse than she'd thought, her daughter wouldn't live another two weeks, and nothing could be done. The damage was irreversible and increasing even faster than expected, in fact faster than this specialist had ever seen. If Miranda didn't act quickly to save her son at the expense of her daughter, she heard, neither twin would reach 24 weeks alive; moreover, even if the boy were rescued, he'd now very likely have severe prematurity problems like blindness, developmental delays or cerebral palsy.

Miranda left the specialist's office with her spirit engulfed by a suffocating darkness. And along the way, she had an epiphany. She remembered that when I'd started her on lipid infusions I'd told her that she'd be kept on these until 12 weeks, and as long as no placenta problems arose, all would be fine. This recollection surged up in her mind with insistent and adamant force. Although it was surrounded by a swirl of emotions, thoughts and images released by the tumult of her enormous stress, this one memory refused to be beaten back into the anonymous depths but persisted in resurfacing to assert itself. She then telephoned me. The conversation is still vivid and fresh to me. She asked me what, in those circumstances, many a doctor might have regarded as a question beyond reason, born out of an instinctive grasping at straws in defiance of all logic and fact. Was there, she demanded, any merit in going back on the lipid infusions? Could it not be that once again her body itself was somehow attacking the placenta and impairing it? And if there was even the slightest possibility of this being so, was there any reason why we shouldn't try what had worked before, albeit in different conditions?

I wished I could encourage her in this line of thought, but, based on all that I knew from the medical literature, I was compelled to admit that I knew of no evidence that lipids would do anything for her endangered twin, since they'd never been used to treat the problem she now faced. I added, though, that since as far as I knew lipid infusions were safe for both mothers and babies, I could present no medical objection against trying them at this stage. In the same breath I begged her not to hold out unreasonable hope as there was also no medical evidence to expect anything to come of it. She seized on my answer enthusiastically and, confirming that she understood and accepted my inability to promise anything, she agreed that this understanding would form the basis of a resumption of the lipid treatment.

Miranda was herself a medical professional. She worked as a physician assistant, a job requiring a highly regulated training that equips graduates to apply for a license to diagnose and to provide treatment, including prescription medicines. Physician assistants are recognized as one of the three professions providing primary medical care, alongside physicians and nurse practitioners. I tell you this to emphasize how heavy Miranda's heart was, because when a layperson with no medical knowledge receives bad news from doctors, it's unsurprising for them to wonder whether the news may be mistaken. If one has no expert knowledge to use in evaluating the news, there always seems a glimmer of a chance, however slender, that the facts may have been erroneously interpreted. In this way, ignorance has an element of bliss in it. But when the bad news is grounded on facts of which you happen to have expert professional knowledge, as Miranda did in this case, and, if on the basis of all your education, those facts appear to make sense, then there is no room for hope unless it comes as a miracle.

The lipid treatment was resumed. Miranda proceeded with a consuming fatigue, and so unrelenting was the outlook that, despite her earlier certainty that losing her little girl was something she could never accept, both she and her husband were now worn down to the ends of their resources, and by the following week they finally accepted, with unspeakable grief, that they had run out of options, and that it seemed their ailing daughter would have to be sacrificed to save her healthy brother.

When they drove to my rooms, this paralyzing prospect oppressed each of them as a burden of mountainous proportions. Miranda wept all the way and they asked the ultrasound technician to shut the patient's viewing screen off because they didn't want to see the baby any more.

After the ultrasound examination, Miranda's husband asked whether anything new was visible. The technician was non-committal and disappeared to fetch me. While they waited, a feeling of inevitability settled on the couple. They'd previously asked what was involved in terminating a twin, and they'd heard how potassium was injected into the baby's heart, stopping it immediately. How awful a thing to contemplate now.

I came into the room and stared at the ultrasound screen silently for about 15 minutes, while the eyes of Miranda and her husband remained fixed on me expectantly. Miranda later said she thought I was quiet for so long because the baby had died. However, I was speechless because I realized I was experiencing a profoundly important moment in medical history. I turned to the couple and said: "It's hard for me to believe what I see. In all my years of practice I have never, ever seen this happen before. Your placenta is functioning normally."

They were stunned. Were they misunderstanding? Miranda murmured: "What did you just say?" I repeated myself, this time with tears in my eyes. Beyond scientific expectation, the damaged placenta had recovered. For the first time since the problem had been detected, the impaired twin's umbilical artery had regained diastolic blood flow, a sign of expanding placenta circulation.

On seeing this on the ultrasound screen, I'd first thought it was a false reading, perhaps a technological glitch. Then, when I saw it was real, I feared the recovery was temporary and would soon reverse itself. But no! Within a week, the blood flow improved further. A week later it moved into normal range. Still better was that the baby's weight improved, reaching the low normal range. Indisputably, the resumed lipid treatment was working.

Miranda's treatment and close monitoring continued, particularly focusing on placenta blood flow, and especially on both twins' brains. After 30 weeks, the little girl started losing some ground again but remained in normal range. By week 33, the babies were given steroids to improve their lung function, and 48 hours later (the time steroids take to work fully) both were delivered. They were small but robust enough not to need breathing aid. They greeted the world in fine voice.

This case shows how a mother can participate proactively in her pregnancy's care. It also illustrates why doctors must listen to patients' instincts about their own bodies. Furthermore, it highlights the value of calculated risks, of keeping an open mind, and of willingness to explore beyond convention. In my experience, the use of lipid infusions this late in a pregnancy was unknown before Miranda's case. Its use here was groundbreaking. Since then I've delivered other healthy babies using this method, including a case where a prestigious hospital told the mother, as Miranda had been told, that she'd have to lose one twin to save the other. Miranda's decision gave her babies their lives as well as a cause for great pride in future: the knowledge that their mother's brave choice not only saved them but has gone on to save others too, and will continue to do so!

We see here the good that can come out of a mother's determination to take ownership of her pregnancy, and from learning as much as possible about the physiology of her womb. Pregnancy complications are physiological, but you needn't be a physician to engage them informedly. Although Miranda had received medical training, she was not an obstetrician or even a doctor; she was an intelligent mother who was deeply committed to understanding everything she could about her pregnancy and its problems. If you have enough of a thirst for knowledge to read this book, you too can acquire enough knowledge to take ownership of your pregnancy. If ever there was an area of human life where knowledge is power, it's the placental aspect of pregnancy!

And this brings us back to the question: where does placenta knowledge come from? The answer may surprise you.

Chapter 11

YOUR PLACENTA AS A COMPUTER SYSTEM

Much of our most generally available information about the placenta doesn't come from studying human pregnancies. We get it from studying pregnant animals, like mice. These studies are useful, but of course animals differ from people. The trouble is that studies of the differences tend to get published in journals aimed at research scientists, not physicians. Few obstetricians read them. They have neither the training nor the time. Consequently, most obstetricians and even high-risk pregnancy specialists have considerable gaps in their detailed placenta knowledge. This is one of the reasons ultrasound is so important. Skilled use of ultrasound can help doctors make up, to some extent, for their knowledge gaps. This can save many babies from death or from lifelong physical and/or mental disability.

The knowledge gaps I'm talking about concern the complexity of placenta activity, especially its highly interactive nature. For many years the placenta was seen as a passive gatekeeper, allowing welcome substances to reach the fetus and waste matter to leave it.

We now know it's more like the center of an elaborate, massively sophisticated computer system whose processes are as crucial to life and safety as those of an air traffic control headquarters at an international airport. Here are some facts that will help you understand this complexity.

Earlier I noted that until about the 10th or 11th week of pregnancy, the mother's blood doesn't even enter the intervillous space to carry nutrients to the baby. Instead, the fetus is nourished mostly by the yolk sac and gland secretions. In this period, the villi have only limited blood vessels. After week 11 or so, villi blood vessel development accelerates and the walls between the maternal and fetal blood get thinner, enabling exchanges of nutrients, oxygen, carbon dioxide and fetal waste. After 12 weeks, spiral artery remodeling goes full blast until it's complete around week 24. Beyond that, the placenta improves mainly in two ways. First, the blood vessels grow enormously in size and number. If you were to lay all the placenta's blood vessel walls flat, at 28 weeks they'd measure about 50 square feet, but in the last 12 weeks they'd measure double that. This is because your baby's weight triples between 28 and 40 weeks, putting an enormous strain on the placenta.

The second way the placenta improves after Week 24 involves not a gain in mass but a loss. The membrane separating maternal and fetal blood, the syncytium, thins down tremendously, losing about five-sixths of its thickness, easing the transfer of substances between the mother's blood and the baby's.

Placenta transfers between mother and fetus happen in different ways. In endocytosis the cargo is sealed in a cyst, or little pouch, that travels through the placental membrane and fastens itself on the destination wall before opening to release the cargo to the fetus. In reverse, when cargo is taken away from the fetus, it's called exocytosis.

A cargo's means of transport through the placental barrier membrane depends on its ability to dissolve in water or fat. The membrane is fatty, so fat-soluble substances are easily transferable.

If all's well by week 24, the placenta can feed the baby all the nutrients it needs. If not, the baby is at risk of problems including pre-eclampsia, overall growth retardation, preterm birth, cerebral palsy, poor brain development, other developmental delays and even death (before or after birth).

We're not sure how different degrees of placenta damage relate to different illnesses, but any damage is bad. A blood clot causing five centimeters (about two inches) of placenta damage can cause retarded growth, hypoxia (oxygen deprivation) and death. A healthy placenta needs enough nutrients and oxygen not only to sustain the baby but also to keep itself running smoothly.

A normal placenta has almost 50% reserve capacity, which means a baby can sometimes survive even if half the placenta is damaged. The question is, in what condition? Acute damage to the placenta tends to be more dangerous and more likely to kill the baby than slow damage over time. Although a baby can survive a significant time without nutrients, oxygen deprivation is another story. If the placenta stops providing enough oxygen, the baby can live only up to ten minutes.

Although oxygen is transferred directly into the fetus's blood, since the womb is a fluid environment, not an air-breathing one, your unborn baby makes motions as if it's breathing, to prepare for its life after birth. As early as 12 to 14 weeks, ultrasound can show its chest expanding and contracting. Instead of air, amniotic fluid, which fills the womb, rushes in and out of its lungs, but no oxygen is delivered in these practice movements. The placenta must supply all the oxygen the baby needs.

Each time you breathe, you suck a mouthful of air into your windpipe. It goes down into your lungs, where its oxygen is transferred to some of your red blood cells. These cells travel to your heart, which (as we saw on our submarine ride) in turn shoots the oxygen-bearing red cells through your bloodstream down to the placenta. There, each red cell gives up its bundle of oxygen, which crosses the placental barrier membrane to be picked up by one of your baby's own red blood cells. The oxygen is propelled through the membrane by the difference in oxygen pressure between your blood vessels and your baby's. The pressure in your baby's vessels is a quarter of the pressure in yours, and any liquid or gas under pressure flows to where there's less pressure. This pressure-driven transfer method helps a baby to cope up to a point with changes in its mother's blood flow when, for example, her blood pressure varies, or when her activities or body position affect her circulation.

The placenta has a similarly amazing way to transport glucose, one of the most basic forms of sugar, across the placental barrier. The ease with which glucose slips through the barrier is almost 50 times higher than we'd generally expect in chemical behavior of this kind, and we don't yet understand exactly how the placenta confers this unusual "power" on glucose in these circumstances. It seems to involve a special protein molecule called a "transporter." There's an important relationship between the baby's intakes of glucose and oxygen. Because oxygen is needed to burn up the glucose for energy, its supply of glucose must be carefully matched to its supply of oxygen. If it has too much glucose and too little oxygen, the glucose gets processed in a way that creates lactic acid (milk acid), and too much of this is dangerous to the baby. This way of processing the glucose also produces much less energy. (It's like making a fire with dry wood, which efficiently gives you a smokeless fire, whereas burning wet wood creates lots of smoke and little warmth.) Adults and babies alike need glucose, but your baby can get by with glucose levels so low that if they happened in an adult bloodstream we'd pass out and might die.

The placenta also controls the cross-membrane transfer of amino acids. These substances, the building-blocks of protein, are like all-purpose chemical bricks that get used to build all sorts of things in the womb. A poor amino acid supply will therefore obstruct your baby's development, with long-term effects. But here's a really astonishing fact: remember how we explained that oxygen gets propelled across the placental membrane by pressure, because the mother's oxygen pressure is higher than the baby's? Well, with amino acids, the pressure works in the opposite direction. Your baby's umbilical cord has a higher blood concentration of amino acids than you do, which means getting amino acids from your blood into your baby's is like getting water to flow uphill. And yet it happens! For this purpose, the placenta again seems to use those mysterious "transporter" molecules. It regulates the activity of these molecules depending on the amino acid levels it senses.

But a fetus can use amino acids only if its general growth rate is healthy to begin with. If its growth is slowed down for any reason, its ability to process amino acids is weakened, no matter how good the fresh supplies are. In one study, increased protein intake to treat fetal growth retardation just made the problem worse. This shows that the placenta isn't just a passive gatekeeper but a sensitive instrument whose complex job is to maintain a subtle balance in your baby's life support system via a variety of mechanisms.

Another important part of this life support system is the group of substances called lipids, which as we've seen are different types of fat. It's not good to be too fat or to eat too much fat, but fat of the right kind, in the right amount, is essential: our bodies use it for building and for energy storage. Fetuses need lipids from Day One of their development. Again, most of what we know about fat transfer across the placental barrier comes from studying animals, not humans, so we must draw conclusions carefully. While a healthy baby produces fatty acids by itself in the last part of pregnancy, a fetus can't produce all the kinds of fatty acid it needs. Some kinds must be obtained from the mother by transfer across the placental barrier.

As is known to anyone who's ever washed dishes, fat doesn't dissolve easily. Bits of fat are thus carried through your bloodstream in little bundles. These come in two kinds. One is called free fatty acids because they float around more or less unattached. The other kind of fat bundle is a lipoprotein, which is basically some fat stuck to a protein molecule. Although we don't understand fully how fats are transferred across the placental barrier, we do know that when free fatty acids reach the barrier they arrive attached to bits of albumin, the main protein found in blood plasma. To get across the barrier, the free fatty acids must be unfastened from the albumin and attached to different transporter proteins. Once they're across the barrier they're then unfastened from the transporter proteins and attached to fetal plasma proteins. The fat molecules that cross the barrier quickest tend to be of a certain size that the placenta senses as being just right; bigger and smaller molecules take longer to gain admission, the way certain travelers get delayed at borders by customs officials while other travelers get easily waved through.

After about 30 weeks, the fastest-growing tissue in the baby's body is fat. At birth, your baby will be converting 90% of its energy intake into fat deposits (some 7000 milligrams a day). All this fat is well used. Your baby's brain and nervous system contain a lot of fatty acids. Because the brain grows fastest in the last 12 weeks, healthy brain development during this period demands a proper supply of essential fatty acids like Omega-6 and Omega-3. To give your baby what it needs, you must eat one molecule of Omega-3 fatty acid for every one to three molecules of Omega-6 fatty acid. In late pregnancy, however, the most popular type of contemporary American diet can't meet the fetal demand for Omega-3 fatty acids: America is afflicted by serious malnutrition as a result of poor dietary education and eating habits. Our highly processed foods result in our tending to eat, on average, 15 to 20 molecules of Omega-6 for every molecule of Omega-3. This severely unhealthy ratio is largely responsible for the explosion of dangerous medical conditions in Western societies, including obesity, diabetes, hypertension and infertility.

Throughout your pregnancy, and preferably even before you become pregnant, you should eat healthy whole foods and avoid highly processed foods. A Mediterranean diet rich in natural vegetables, olive oil and fish, with limited meat and animal fat, can make a profound difference to your baby's brain development, nervous system development and general health. If necessary, take Omega-3 supplements. Omega-3 is in fish, but seafood now contains so many cancer-causing substances (because of pollution) that eating fish more than twice a week isn't healthy. Ask your doctor to supply you with a healthy fish oil supplement.

Which brings us to metals. Believe it or not, your placenta also transfers across its membrane barrier various metals including molybdenum and manganese. In extremely small quantities, these trace elements are vital to adults, children and unborn babies alike. A copper deficiency, for example, can lead to a variety of illnesses including blood vessel disorders. Too little selenium can affect thyroid functioning, leading to brain problems and repeated miscarriages. Insufficient iron can cause anemia and death. Poor levels of zinc can cause several kinds of sickness. Some investigators have associated trace element deficiencies with impaired fetal development and variations in birth weight and size, including head circumference. The role of trace elements again illustrates the importance of placenta monitoring to maintain the right balance of substances to meet fetal needs. Some trace elements are indispensable for survival, yet too much of them can poison your baby. [48-58]

Chapter 12

EVERYTHING YOU LET INTO YOUR BODY AFFECTS YOUR BABY'S CHANCES

A vital fact in understanding your placenta's role is that everything you eat, drink or otherwise take into your body can affect your baby's health and even its chances of making it to full term. That includes drugs of any kind, some of which can cross the barrier very quickly. The old belief that no drugs used by a mother could penetrate the placental barrier was shattered in the 1960s when the morning-sickness drug thalidomide was shown to be responsible for severe birth defects. Despite this tragic experience, improved safety and selectivity of drug therapy in pregnancy continue not to be a universal priority in drug design and development. To my perception, the pharmaceutical industry tends to sidestep much responsibility for the effects of drug use in pregnancy. You, as a mother, have to look out for your baby in this regard. You need to recognize that any substance you let into your body both during and preceding pregnancy has the potential to cross the placental barrier to at least some extent and get into your baby.

Drug-affected birth defects can especially take shape in the first three months, when the liver, brain, heart and other key organs are being formed. During pregnancy, therefore, you should use drugs only when they're essential. This might sound obvious, but because current knowledge indicates that most medical prescription drugs are generally safe in this respect, physicians tend to be concerned with the congenital defect potential of only a few drugs. Nevertheless, in certain circumstances epigenetic effects on fetal DNA, which I discussed in previous pages, can profoundly influence fetal physiology in ways that may not show up until decades into adulthood.[59-65] It is very important for you to make sure your doctor is familiar with these possibilities, which can be associated not only with drugs but also with chemical products used in farming, the food industry, packaging, cosmetic products, artificial sweeteners and other kinds of manufacturing. Such epigenetic changes can occur before you conceive as well as during pregnancy. Your rule of thumb should be: ingest only substances that will benefit you and your baby with minimal, if not zero, side effects.

Also important in this context is your body's defense system, aspects of which I've explained earlier. Some of this system's white blood cells produce antibodies (also called immunoglobulins): protein molecules shaped like a Y. Each kind of antibody is specialized to latch on to a specific enemy of your body, such as a certain kind of germ. By doing this it disables the germ or, if it can't, it at least serves to mark the germ so it be clearly sensed and shot down by the rest of your body's defenses. Whether an antibody can cross the placental barrier depends on when the mother's body starts manufacturing that type of antibody. If a pregnant mother is struck by an infection she's never had before, so that she starts manufacturing antibodies against that infection for the very first time after her pregnancy has begun, those antibodies won't have chemical visas to cross the placental barrier and therefore won't be able to protect the baby. However, if the mother was exposed to that infection (say, hepatitis B) before she became pregnant, then when she's exposed to it again during pregnancy her body will already have in place a process to manufacture those specific antibodies in a form which, being familiar to the body, will automatically be allowed through the placental barrier to protect the baby.

There are five main sorts of antibodies. The most common, and also the smallest, is the only type that can cross the placental barrier, and its working life lasts about three months. As delivery approaches, your body's highest concentration of these antibodies will be in your baby's blood. They'll defend your baby for at least three months after birth, by which time a healthy baby's immune system should start producing its own antibodies. Your newborn may even continue to receive some support from your antibodies up to six months, especially if you breast feed.

Antibodies are very important to your baby both before and after birth. Repeated infections can confuse the immune system, triggering the production of antibodies that attack the body's own tissues. Chronic autoimmune disorders can develop as a result.

Among other bad effects, infection in a newborn baby can stunt growth. We're not sure how this happens, but it's reasonable to theorize that if the baby channels too much of its precious energy into fighting infection, it has less energy for growth. Recent experiments with ducks have shown that infections not only changed the ducks' bodies and energy levels dramatically, but shortened their lives. As I've mentioned, information from studies of animals must be assessed carefully to determine its applicability to people. But it's always worth thinking about if only because it can open up new trains of thought that indeed have human relevance.

Given these facts about infection, it follows that although you need to exercise extreme caution about what you take into your body during pregnancy, it's vital to strike a wise balance with this. You and your baby must receive the support of medications if and when this becomes appropriate. The cases I've already described to you illustrate the great difference that can be made by the timely administration of appropriate medication. Even when medication comes with risks, the potential benefits may outweigh the potential dangers. Drugs are listed in categories according to the risks they pose, and drugs that offer significant risks which can be outweighed by their potential benefits are in Category D. One of the situations where medication is needed despite some risk is in premature labor. As I explained earlier, by using nifedipine and indomethacin, two uterus muscle relaxants, my clinic prevented prematurity in 90% of patients who went into premature labor. Another instance where timely medication may be needed is heart disease (whose medical name, cardiovascular disease, is more accurate because it isn't just about the heart; it's also about the blood vessels, hence the "vascular"). This disease is commonly thought of as an ailment of nervous middle-aged men who smoke and who eat too many cheeseburgers, but this stereotype is misleading. Heart disease is a major cause of death among pregnant mothers and unborn babies. One of its features, hypertension, complicates up to 15% of pregnancies. Pregnant women with heart disease are at risk of death. They face heart failure, arrhythmias (irregular heartbeats), stroke (interrupted blood flow causing a sudden breakdown in brain function), and a serious weakening of the heart muscle in late pregnancy or within a few months after birth. Babies whose mothers have heart disease are at risk of growth restriction, premature birth and death.

One of the most frequently used heart disease drugs is digoxin, which comes from the foxglove plant, digitalis. A drug called a beta-blocker is also commonly used for pregnant mothers with hypertension and arrhythmia. Some cells in your body, in the heart and elsewhere, have special parts called beta receptors, which are like panic buttons that sound an alarm when they sense that something stressful is happening. These receptors can be over-sensitive, though, resulting in inappropriately raised levels of stress, so the beta-blocker drug numbs them to give you some peace. The safety of beta-blockers for pregnant mothers and their babies seems to depend on when in the pregnancy you take them. Taking them in the second three months of pregnancy is associated with reduced fetal and placental growth. When they're taken in the last three months, only the placenta's weight seems affected. We're unsure whether these problems come from the beta-blocker itself or from the hypertension or other heart disease that the beta-blocker is treating. Evidence so far indicates that, in this case, the heart disease is the culprit, not the drug.

We also sometimes have to use anticonvulsant drugs. Epilepsy is the most common neurological (nervous system) disorder in pregnancy, affecting up to one in 100 expectant mothers. When people say their nerves are frayed, or something is getting on their nerves, they're usually referring to their state of mind, but of course the nervous system isn't limited to our thoughts and feelings: a vast network of nerve tissues extends throughout our bodies, forming the communication system by which the various parts of the body talk to each other. If something goes seriously wrong with our nervous system it can be as disastrous as a major computer crash. An epileptic seizure is pretty much a biological counterpart of a computer crash; it involves a kind of power surge or burst of abnormal electrical activity in the brain. Some (though not all) seizures result in abnormal signals being sent out through the nervous system, causing muscles to tighten and relax intermittently in the phenomenon we call a convulsion. During pregnancy you must do everything you can to avoid a seizure, which can seriously damage both you and your baby. The effects can include placental abruption (where the placenta lining tears loose from the uterus), fetal hypoxia (oxygen deprivation), bleeding in the brain and increased risk of fetal deformity.

A big problem in dealing with seizures is that anticonvulsant drugs are themselves associated with risks of deformities or poisoning. In general, for instance, if you take the drug valproate during pregnancy, your baby's risk of major birth defects is multiplied more than five times.[66, 67] But this statistic must be placed in careful perspective and shouldn't be used simplistically as the basis of a medical decision because as scary as it sounds, it's balanced by the equally important fact that most babies aren't harmed by valproate. Although there's statistical risk, valproate should be used if the mother needs it because the dangers from repeated seizures are worse than the risks of any conventional anti-epileptic medication. But if you need an anti-seizure medication, make sure you receive the one that's best for your disorder, as prescribed by your neurologist.

The difference between problems of the nervous system, such as epilepsy, and the psychological problems that most people mean when they speak about their nerves being worn out, doesn't mean psychological problems deserve less attention. On the contrary: sometimes medication is certainly needed to treat them. But here again, great care must be taken to ensure that such medicine serves the best interests of both mother and baby. For example, pregnant mothers commonly become temporarily depressed: antidepressants are among the most widely prescribed Category D drugs during pregnancy. The trouble is, most antidepressant drugs can affect the formation of the fetal nervous system. This can in turn harm the baby's ability to develop normal behavior patterns. An example is the type of drug called an SSRI (selective serotonin reuptake inhibitors, serotonin being a neurotransmitter, a chemical used by our nervous system to transmit signals). Newborns who've been exposed to this type of drug in the womb are less active than they should be in the first few days of their lives, with abnormally low pulse rates and abnormalities in their facial expressions, breathing and ability to control the movement of their bodies. Controversial recent findings suggest that some SSRI medications might be responsible for a congenital heart defect, pulmonary stenosis.[68-70] The long-term side effects of SSRI medicines aren't yet known. This needs to be balanced against the fact that if a pregnant mother is significantly depressed or stressed this can be worse for the unborn than any known harm from currently common antidepressant drugs. Maternal stress has been associated with potentially dangerous pregnancy complications as well as impairment of the baby's ability to manage stress in childhood and adulthood.

We must now come back to HIV (human immunodeficiency

virus), the cause of AIDS (acquired immunodeficiency syndrome), which I mentioned briefly when discussing antiviral drugs. Having sketched a picture for you of how drugs relate to the placenta,

I need to say more about HIV. Almost 18 million women worldwide are HIV-positive, i.e. they have this virus in them. Many people are HIV-positive without knowing it. In some areas almost 30 out of every 100 pregnant women will have HIV. Some 90% of all children who develop HIV get it from their mothers in the womb. But the good news is that there's a very good chance of protecting the baby if the right antiviral drugs are used. If such drugs are needed, they must be used during pregnancy and labor as well as after the baby is born. Using a combination of drugs to protect a baby in this situation seems to work better against HIV than using just a single drug.

It's easy to become confused about whether prescription drugs are good or bad in pregnancy. While few, if any, drugs are ever free of risks, most prescription drugs tend to be acceptably safe for pregnancy, provided the prescription is a sound response to the messages that mother and doctor are receiving from the womb, the placenta and the mother's physiological system. Always ask your doctor exactly why he or she is prescribing a medication, what it's expected to do, and what risk it poses for the baby. Generally, a responsible, competent physician will prescribe a medication on a trade-off basis, whereby the risks are balanced against the expected or hoped-for benefits. But it's always your right (and responsibility) as a mother to ask for explanations to reassure you that a medicine is acceptably safe for the baby in the context of the reason for its prescription. With the many drugs now available, most maternal illnesses during pregnancy can be effectively treated without significant or unwarranted risk to the baby. [71]

Chapter 13

THINGS THAT CAN GO WRONG...

So I've given you examples of the kinds of things that can go wrong with pregnancy, especially as far as the placenta is concerned, and I've mentioned quite a few other potential problems in passing. We now need to look at these potential problems more closely. Before I move on to that, though, this is a good time to make a few other points that I believe you'll find helpful.

The old saying "blood is thicker than water" (i.e. family ties tend to be more important to people than just about anything else) is a good introduction to these points since they involve water, blood and a bit more about the basis of family ties: genes.

We all have a lot more water in us than blood. In fact, blood itself, as well as almost everything else inside us, is mainly made of water. Water accounts for some 90% of a fetus's weight and about 60% of an average adult's: our entire bodies are made up largely of fluids. Cerebrospinal fluid, which cushions your brain in your skull and is also found inside the brain as well as in the spinal cord, is some 99% water. Your blood plasma is over 90% water and your urine over 95%. The fluid between and within your body's cells is largely made of water, as is the amniotic fluid that fills the amniotic sac in which your fetus lives until birth. Water is so omnipresent in your body that it's misleading to think of it as an ingredient; it's more accurate to see your body as an arrangement of different amounts of water varying in concentration from place to place and from organ to organ. In view of this, it seems only logical that our bodies are designed for water to have a kind of free pass for movement in your body. No membranes turn it away. A molecule of water could move from the tip of your toe to the tip of your finger without any road blocks along the way. This isn't just a figure of speech. It's been observed in studies where water molecules have been labeled with radioactivity and then followed as they moved freely and swiftly through the body. Wherever such a molecule traveled it would be greeted by familiar water-based objects and environments. In a sense, the water in your body is continuous: one water molecule after another. Every water molecule is linked to every other one by all the water molecules in between them. Fetal tissue growth needs a constant supply of water during the entire pregnancy, and as with other fetal demands your water intake must be constant but just right; neither too much nor too little. The process by which water moves through membranes is called diffusion. Water in the placenta moves both between and through the cells; the placenta's job includes transferring enough water at just the right rate.

The placenta's role in maintaining an optimal rate of water transfer is mirrored by its roles in controlling and adjusting the supply to the fetus of other vital substances. While some of these substances come to the placenta from elsewhere in the body, some are manufactured by the placenta itself. One of its tasks is to serve as a gland, a "factory" organ that makes and secretes substances like hormones, the signaling chemicals that trigger or effect changes in various parts of the body, including chemical processes and states which combine physical sensations with emotional responses like hunger, fear and sexual stimulation. The placenta produces hormones that are essential to fetal development. Some of these hormones even do the work that would normally be done by a nervous system, which, in the early stages of pregnancy, your fetus hasn't yet had time to form. Some placenta hormones also regulate the secretions of other placenta hormones. And during pregnancy the placenta is your body's main source of estrogens, the main female sex hormones that create attributes we associate with female-ness. In non-pregnant women, estrogens are produced by the ovaries; during pregnancy their production is taken over by the placenta. Another hormone produced exclusively by the placenta is HCG (human chorionic gonadotropin), which is needed for the secretion of another hormone, progesterone, during pregnancy's first three months. Progesterone gives the uterus a thick lining of blood vessels and capillaries to sustain the growing fetus.

All the physiological functions described above are in turn regulated by genes. Though I discussed genes earlier, I must now add a crucial point about them. It's commonly believed that if you have good genes all will be well with your pregnancy. Not so. Even the best genes can't guarantee a successful pregnancy if you have a weak placenta, which can weaken for reasons that have little to do with genes. Paradoxically, despite the placenta's formidable strengths, it's enormously sensitive, because great complexity brings vulnerability. I don't exaggerate when I tell you that the number of perfectly normal placentas I've seen can be counted on the fingers of one hand.

How, then, is it possible for most babies that make it to delivery to be born healthy? Because the placenta is programmed to grow with excess capacity to compensate for abnormalities. This alone is cause for courage in the face of placental problems. But, as I've explained, we can't rely on placental resilience to fix everything. There are crises that the placenta can't handle without help. If one of these strikes, encouraging statistics about placental resilience won't change the fact that you'll be concerned not with most pregnancies but with your own.

On, now, to the kinds of crises that can occur. Earlier, I described the normal placenta as shaped somewhat like a round loaf joined to a cord (the umbilical cord) containing one umbilical vein, which brings oxygenated blood and nutrients from the placenta to the baby, plus two umbilical arteries via which the baby sends waste and deoxygenated blood to the placenta. The length of the umbilical cord is proportional to fetal activity. Most cords are 1 to 1½ centimeters thick (i.e. ⅓ to about ½ inch) and about 50 centimeters (20 inches) long. When the cord is less than 30 centimeters (just about 12 inches), the risk of cord accident and fetal loss increases significantly. Ideally, the cord is attached to the very center of the placenta but sometimes it's off-center. It can even connect to the placenta's edge. The worst is when it misses the placenta entirely and attaches in the amniotic membranes. This is very bad; the fetus can suffer severe growth restriction and may die. Then there's eccentric cord insertion, when it joins between the edge of the placental disk and the center. This happens in about 25 in 100 pregnancies and is serious, not because of the position of the cord, but because of the circumstances that caused it. These kinds of cord abnormalities are more likely with twins or more.

We've seen how the spot where the embryo implants itself in the uterus is the center of what will become the placenta. The normal placenta takes shape around that spot concentrically, in the form of an expanding circle radiating outward. If the circle's expansion is impeded on one side, the placenta grows in one direction, leaving the cord in a lopsided or eccentric position. Something similar can happen later in pregnancy if part of the placenta is afflicted by abnormal blood-clotting which causes the affected tissues to wither. If this happens early, the placenta can partly compensate for it, but if it happens later it's a bigger problem. To enable any necessary treatment to be given in good time, the placental cord position should be checked by ultrasound throughout the pregnancy. If, at any time, the cord is found to be eccentric, the placenta must be examined for areas of abnormal clotting damage, which can be treated, as we'll see. Fetal growth should also be monitored with ultrasound every 2 to 4 weeks, depending on the growth rate. It's important to confirm that the cord develops properly, i.e. with two arteries plus a vein). If there's no vein, the fetus will die. If there's a vein but just one artery, the result isn't necessarily death but the danger is very great; far greater than that posed by an eccentric cord. Although most babies with a vein and just one artery are born normal, such cords do increase the risk of fetal defects, so if there's any sign of this you must see an experienced perinatologist (specialist in high-risk pregnancies) right away to check for possible fetal defects and to determine the cause. Most two-vessel cords are caused by accident or thrombosis (abnormal clotting). When the cause is thrombosis early in the pregnancy, the lone umbilical artery grows up to $1\frac{1}{2}$ normal size, which can compensate adequately for the missing artery. But thrombosis later in pregnancy can severely restrict fetal growth and the fetus may die.

In most cases where babies die because of two-vessel cords, evidence suggests this is because of insufficient monitoring so that the two-vessel cord isn't detected soon enough to treat.[72] Although better monitoring can't prevent all stillborns, it improves the baby's chances. When placental blood vessel damage due to clotting is detected early enough, extensive clinical experience has shown that treatment can often be very successful, resulting in a healthy birth. I've found Doppler technology to be essential in these situations. Doppler examination doesn't just use ultrasound to create a picture of the baby; it also measures the speed and direction of blood flowing through your blood vessels and your baby's. (It's named after Christian Doppler, a 19th-century Austrian who first worked out this kind of calculation.) So, if your doctor thinks you may have a 2-vessel cord, ask right away to be expertly checked for placental damage.[73, 74] Your blood may also need to be tested for thrombophilia. Whatever the results, all 2-vessel-cord mothers should take a baby aspirin (81 milligrams) a day to minimize further clotting damage. If thrombophilia is found, you'll need appropriate anticoagulant treatment.

If you have a two-vessel cord without thrombophilia, the father should be tested for thrombophilia. (Fathers can pass it on to the baby.) If your doctor is reluctant to test, consult another doctor.

Two other placental abnormalities you should know about are placenta previa and vasa previa. In placenta previa (the Latin previa means "in the way"), the placenta forms in an abnormal place, namely the lowest part of the uterus. Because of this location, it blocks the internal cervical os, which is the opening of the birth canal. The placenta should be in the upper part of the uterus, leaving the birth canal open and clear for use as the baby's route to leave your body. In vasa previa, blood vessels get caught between the baby and the opening of the cervix, risking interference with the delivery of oxygen to the baby. Also, rupturing of these mislocated vessels during labor can cause dangerous fetal bleeding and fetal death. The internal cervical os is easy to block, being only a few millimeters (a small fraction of an inch) wide. There are varieties of blockage, e.g.: complete obstruction; implantation of a small part of the placenta in the lower part of the uterus (in these cases the placenta tends to reposition itself to a better location eventually); just the edge of the placenta covering part of the os or bordering it; and low-lying placenta, which isn't placenta previa but can cause similar bleeding problems, especially if the placenta edge is very close to the os (such cases should be managed exactly like placenta previa).

Placenta previa can be predicted. Its signs can be diagnosed in the ninth month in about one in 300 pregnancies. If it happens, a vaginal birth can kill the mother and/or baby, so delivery must be via caesarean section (often called just "a caesarian"), removing the baby through cuts in the tummy and uterus.

I've spoken above of the placenta repositioning itself in the uterus, but this doesn't mean it moves. Wherever it is, it's very much attached. Here's what happens in repositioning. Usually the cervix area isn't rich in blood vessels, and, as we've seen, a rich network of blood vessels is vital to the placenta. So when the placenta forms too near the cervix the part of the placenta that's closest to the cervix usually withers because of its poor access to blood. The placenta then compensates by expanding where there are enough blood vessels. In doing so it effectively repositions itself even though it hasn't detached itself and moved. Heavy bleeding may occur during this repositioning and rebuilding. This can be scary but holds no great danger. I've never seen a baby lost to placenta previa in early pregnancy. The earliest miscarriage I've seen it cause was in a patient with complete previa: at 22 weeks she began bleeding profusely and had to have hysterotomy (early caesarean) to save her life. (This isn't a hysterectomy, or removal of the uterus.)

When placenta previa is diagnosed early, the prevention of excessive bleeding can be helped if you avoid: aspirin, ibuprofen and related non-steroidal anti-inflammatory medications; intercourse; heavy lifting (and anything that can increase abdominal pressure, like constipation); and internal digital vaginal examinations (when the doctor puts a finger into your cervix to evaluate for labor signs). Also, have an ultrasound examination by an experienced obstetrician or ultrasound technologist. It's safe and very important in monitoring this condition.

If placenta previa is diagnosed in the first three months, the previa tissue that caused the obstruction will likely wither away in a few weeks. Ultrasound can help track this so you'll know when it's safe to resume normal activity. If you have placenta previa in late pregnancy, have a caesarean as soon as the baby's complete lung development is confirmed by amniocentesis, an analysis of a small sample of fluid from the amniotic sac, which your doctor will withdraw with a needle. The best time for amniocentesis is usually week 35, when more than 80% of babies are mature. If the results show your baby's lungs aren't ready to breathe, have weekly amniocentesis until you know a caesarean is safe. If you have bleeding or signs of preterm labor, ask your doctor about having amniocentesis sooner or even being delivered immediately, because placenta previa bleeding can be catastrophic to mothers.

Let's now look at the rare condition vasa previa, where blood vessels get caught between the baby and the cervical opening, threatening oxygen flow to the baby and creating a risk of dangerous bleeding if these vessels break during labor. Before we had ultrasound, vasa previa went undetected until blood vessels ruptured, but expertly used ultrasound with Doppler technology can now accurately diagnose almost all vasa previa conditions very early. Any one of various conditions can be associated with vasa previa, including growth in the uterus of an accessory lobe, a "twin" placenta that doesn't develop beyond being a lump of tissue. It tends to appear opposite the real placenta. To nourish the accessory lobe, the blood vessels feeding the placenta put out extensions which form the vasa previa by crossing over the cervix. Vasa previa can also arise from a placenta lying so low in the uterus that the umbilical cord vessels don't join the main placental disk in the normal way but enter the amniotic sac membranes far from the placenta. This is more common in multiple pregnancies. There's no treatment for it, so when it's found, the baby should be delivered by caesarean as soon as lung maturity is confirmed with amniocentesis or sooner if necessary, after your doctor administers corticosteroids to assist the achievement of lung maturity.

An abnormality that affects 1 in 100 pregnancies is placental abruption. Here part of the placenta detaches from its blood vessels and from the uterine wall. There might be a little vaginal bleeding, but the affected part of the placenta tends to be small in relation to the remaining healthy placenta; when there's no bleeding, we usually learn of an abruption by ultrasound or even only after birth. About half of all abruption cases need special care. A third are severe: in half of the severe cases, the babies die and the survivors have a very high incidence of long-term nervous system problems from asphyxia (insufficient oxygen) during birth. Once in every 300 or so pregnancies, we see a severe abruption that can be lethal to both baby and mother and thus needs hospital admission or immediate delivery. If the mother bleeds a lot, it can be easy to diagnose; absent vaginal bleeding, the first sign could be severe abdominal pain, back pain, abdominal tenderness or an abnormal fetal heart rate. Pressing on the uterus hurts, and the uterus may feel hard as a board. Ultrasound can confirm abruption in many cases but not in all, especially if the ultrasound technician is inexperienced. A fresh blood clot reflecting sound waves can look like tissue on the screen, causing many misdiagnoses. Early ultrasound detection of abruption works best if the image shows a very specific telltale sight: a line of compressed tissue that crosses the placenta between the blood clot and the placenta surface in the area of detachment. But recognizing this needs a very experienced eye.[43, 75]

Complicating things further is that severe abruption and its associated conditions can develop so fast there's often no time for ultrasound. The diagnosis must be made instantly on the basis of available information or the baby may die or at least be seriously harmed, so it's preferable to err on the side of caution. Better a healthy baby delivered somewhat early than waiting for certainty at the cost of delivering the baby brain-damaged or dead.

Now, I've said that bleeding needn't be dangerous, but I've also said that bleeding from placenta previa can be catastrophic. These two statements may seem conflictual. In fact, they aren't, and it's important for you to understand why. We're talking about two different situations. In early pregnancy, previa bleeding poses no great threat, whereas bleeding from previa in the second half of the pregnancy or, worse, in the last five 5 to 10 weeks, can be disastrous due to anatomical changes and the size of the mature placental blood vessels. With previa, as with so much else in the placenta's life, there's always a fine line between what we can predict and what surprises even experienced doctors. To illustrate how murky this line can be, let me dip again into my case files and share with you the story of a patient I'll call Shelley.

Chapter 14

SHELLEY'S STORY

When I called up Shelley's case for this book, I seemed to be visiting the home of a normal, healthy family. Shelley and her husband Rand had three robust sons who did all the rowdy things tough boys should be doing. However, things could have been tragically different.

Before their boys arrived this couple struggled with infertility for 2 years. Their anguish was made heavier by Shelley's job as a labor room nurse, constantly holding other women's babies. Then finally, Shelley fell pregnant through IUI (intrauterine insemination). It seemed to her like a miracle. At last, at 29, she had a bump. The day she learned she was expecting a girl, she rushed to buy a few baby clothes and a toy and began decorating the baby's room. Nothing extravagant. Just enough to show the world that she too was going to be a mother. Rand teased his wife that the baby would have a fine voice, like Rand's mother, and they began to refer to their unborn daughter as Lark.

Everything progressed well, and at 12 weeks Shelley went for a routine nuchal translucency (NT) scan, where ultrasound measures the amount of fluid in the fetus's nuchal area (nape of the neck). Down syndrome is associated with a higher volume of fluid. She also had her PAPP-A (pregnancy associated plasma protein A) level tested: a low level can signify an elevated risk of Down syndrome.

The results showed that Lark likely had Down syndrome. Moreover, Rand and Shelley learned they'd have to wait another four weeks for an amniocentesis to confirm this diagnosis since only then would Lark be big enough for amniocentesis to be safe.

They were weeks of agony. Then the amniocentesis was done … and it turned out Lark did not have Down syndrome! The initial test result was due to the phenomenon of false positives. According to a 2012 study published by Professor Jack Canick, of the Warren Alpert Medical School at Brown University, in Providence, Rhode Island, a combination of an NT scan with certain types of biochemical testing can give a false positive result for Down syndrome up to 5% of tests.

Yet this test imperfection wasn't wholly to blame for the weeks of protracted stress that Shelley and Rand had endured. What they didn't know was that amniocentesis wasn't the only way to verify a positive Down syndrome result. Another test was available: chorionic villus sampling (CVS), using a tissue sample from the placenta. A CVS could have been done immediately.

Why wasn't it done in this case? Doctors can choose not to do a CVS for any of several reasons. A CVS requires expertise that not all doctors have. Patients might also hear that a CVS is risky, though modern techniques make this argument questionable.

Shelley later recalled that she wasn't told the CVS option existed. She'd loved to have known about it, not only to avoid the 4 weeks of waiting but because her amniocentesis was a far from good experience. First, it seems that despite the weeks of waiting, she wasn't given a specific appointment for the amniocentesis. She went to her doctor for what she thought was a routine checkup. She wasn't psychologically prepared for an amniocentesis that day, nor had she made arrangements to be driven home from the doctor's office. As a nurse, she knew what the procedure entailed, and it was her understanding that she shouldn't be alone after it. As she later reported it, events unfolded, astonishingly, as follows. She asked if she could reschedule it but was told her doctor was too busy to do it any other time. She then became hysterical and asked for the amniocentesis not to be done, but the doctor called assistants who restrained her as the needle was inserted.

Shelley began to bleed. After more tests, she was told that although Lark didn't have Down syndrome, there was risk of fetal growth retardation, prematurity or death. She couldn't later recollect much being explained to her about this. Her doctor kept monitoring the pregnancy, hoping matters would improve, but she was unaware of any proactive treatment being applied. After the amniocentesis, Shelley went to a high-risk pregnancy specialist who'd once worked with her. His opinion: it didn't look good.

Around week 18, she heard Lark wasn't going to make it. When she talked about this much later, her voice would still become tense with frustration and bewilderment. As she remembered it, she kept hearing "horror stories" with no advice on what to do. She was advised to come in weekly for the next two months. When she asked for an explanation of her condition, the answer was that no explanation was available. The doctor, she would recall, kept telling her: "Miscarriages happen." Appalled, Shelley protested that there was no miscarriage; her baby was still alive inside her. But nobody had an explanation for her.

The next weeks were a blur. She became increasingly depressed, crying almost constantly. Rand was equally devastated. One day later, he phoned her from work. He'd been agonizing over Lark's fate and was adamant that he would not simply wait inactively for catastrophe. A friend of his had given him the name of a doctor whom Shelley must call at once.

Her experience up to then had been such that she saw little point in seeing yet another doctor, and although the doctor Rand was talking about happened to be me, I understand how she felt. After all, she already had a high-risk specialist and no one seemed to know what was going on. Also, it was 6 PM, and she thought, even if she called, no one would pick up. She dialed the number anyway and a voice did answer, and Shelley explained her situation briefly. She was asked to hold on while her summary was relayed to me. With nothing to lose, she waited. After a while, the voice came back and told her the doctor wanted to see her. She assumed this meant she must make an appointment and was surprised to hear that, no, she must come right away. She explained that she lived at least an hour away; she was told I would wait for her. On Shelley's arrival, I conducted an extensive ultrasound evaluation and then asked her to call Rand, who was still at work, an hour away in normal traveling time. But he sped there in 30 minutes. When they were both seated with me, I told them my news.

Severe placental thrombosis had damaged more than half the placenta, which, additionally, was abnormally thick, a condition associated with fetal asphyxia and fetal death. There was no amniotic fluid. Lark must already have suffered brain damage from lack of oxygen. She might have suffered a stroke, which would account for the hydrocephalus (excessive fluid in the brain ventricles) that I'd seen. Further, Shelley's cervix had shortened because her body was rejecting the fetus and reacting against the inflammation produced by the necrotic placenta tissues. To my profound sorrow, I had to tell them that due to all that happened, Lark had no chance. If we didn't end the pregnancy, Shelley's body would. As both she and Rand did what they could to cope with this information, I felt a responsibility to tell them also that if they decided to persist with this pregnancy, and if against all expectations Lark somehow managed to be born alive, she would be seriously impaired, bringing her into a life of tremendous difficulty, and possibly of suffering, not to mention the terrible cost to spirit, mind and body that caring for her would from then on impose on the rest of their lives.

It all looked unbearable until we came to the point in our discussion that changed everything, when, specifically addressing Shelley, I told her that when the ordeal of this pregnancy was over, she must take three months off and then conceive again, and I made her this promise: "As long as there are no genetic problems, I guarantee you a healthy baby." I added that I planned to make good on this promise by devoting myself to the care of Shelley's placenta.

As a nurse, Shelley appreciated the placenta's importance, but my promise nevertheless seemed hard to believe, and again I could well understand this. She wasn't even sure she could conceive again. She'd been told repeatedly she'd never have children, so her conceiving at all had seemed miraculous. Now she had to start all over again? Despite their stress, the couple decided in three days. I'd explained that beyond 21 weeks there'd have to be a vaginal birth and this Shelley didn't want. With difficulty they found a doctor willing to end so advanced a pregnancy, and it was done while she was asleep. The hardest part was returning home to a nursery she'd prepared against Rand's warning. Even more traumatic was that four days later her milk came. The distraught Rand locked himself in the nursery and wept.

As I'd suggested, they waited 3 months before returning to her fertility doctor to try to conceive anew. The initial round of IUI failed, but on the very day of Lark's expected birth, Shelley conceived. While she understood that a different life now stirred in her, it felt like a continuation of Lark's story. She immediately placed herself under my clinic's intensive care. Blood tests showed both parents had thrombophilia: three maternal genetic mutations; one paternal. Their baby would have at least one genetic mutation and at most three. A treatment plan was devised to keep her placenta healthy. Long afterwards, Shelley could still reel the plan off: vitamin B, aspirin, enoxaparin sodium, metformin for 12 weeks, detailed ultrasounds every two weeks. At first, with images of Lark's sonograms vivid in her mind, she approached the ultrasound appointments with dread, but her fears soon dissipated. She prayed for a healthy baby. After a relatively uncomplicated 38-week pregnancy, she and Rand had a bonny son, Alan.

After 10 months, Shelley conceived again, this time without trying! After 9 months of close monitoring and pre-emptive perinatological treatment, a healthy second son, Marcus, arrived. The story still wasn't over, though. To the couple's surprise, a third conception followed, delivering another healthy boy, Ben. This story offers much food for thought. Lark's problems resulted directly in Shelley's receiving appropriate placental diagnosis and treatment. If this hadn't happened when it did, Lark could have been born dead, or alive with severe handicaps, with the medical issues remaining undiagnosed and untreated. Shelley's subsequent babies could then have been born with serious physical and mental handicaps caused by her continuing untreated problems. Although her first pregnancy ended with grief, her three sons almost certainly owed their good health to their lost sister. The only assuredly better scenario would have been if events had steered Shelley earlier to receive the examinations that identified her medical issues and saved the little girl with the same treatment that gave good health to her brothers. But it's needlessly tormenting to contemplate what-ifs beyond a point. I believe the wise perspective on Shelley's case is to reflect on what it tells us about the delicate balance between a healthy and unhealthy placenta. Further, it eloquently illustrates how warning signs from a distressed placenta can be overlooked. Medical professionals can mistakenly dismiss danger signs like early evidence of abnormally low **PAPP-A**, sporadic bleeding, fetal hydrocephalus (which is too often labeled a genetic mystery instead of being seen in a placenta-related context) and clotting damage due to thrombophilia. When I first read Shelley's case history, I saw no mention of any ultrasound examination of the placenta. This doesn't mean fingers should be pointed at any individual doctors; inadequate placental monitoring has become such a common part of established medical culture that it can be very uncomfortable for doctors to deviate from this tendency of their peers. In the prior case histories of the many patients who have come to my clinic when their pregnancies reached crisis point, I've found information on the condition of the placenta to be rare if not wholly absent. Another useful aspect of Shelley's case is that it illustrates chorionic villus sampling (CVS). In the 1980s, doctors would mainly do transcervical CVS procedures, where a catheter is inserted through the vagina to secure a sample of placental tissue for analysis. Since then, a transabdominal CVS has been developed, in which the sample is secured by inserting a needle through the abdomen and uterus. (My co-researchers K D'Amico, T McGuiness, D Clay, and K King and I published a paper on this in 1995.)[76] Clinical experience has shown that an expertly done transabdominal CVS is safer than amniocentesis, and, in cases like Shelley's, it can be done without the delay that she and Rand were made to go through. Overall, then, while Shelley and Rand went through some horrible experiences their story overall offers encouragement and hope to all mothers facing pregnancy complications. While I was working on this book, Shelley recalled that after losing her first baby many women, including Rand's grandmother, had told her they too had suffered miscarriages, sometimes without anyone else knowing because it often isn't something people want to talk about. She reported that Lark remained present to her and Rand, as they understood she'd helped them have their boys. She added that after I'd promised that with the right treatments, she'd definitely have a beautiful, healthy child, she'd gone back to her obgyn and told him. His answer was a derisive laugh...

Chapter 15

TESTING, TIMING, PREVENTION

You'll remember that severe placental thrombosis damaged more than half of Shelley's placenta, that her unborn baby was brain-damaged from lack of oxygen, and had probably suffered a stroke due to thrombophilia. I've explained that preventing such outcomes requires taking action early enough rather than waiting for a crisis. Timing is the key to many if not all the pregnancy problems discussed in this book. Some of my patients have come to think of their successful escape from their pregnancy complications as miraculous, but the clinical professionals involved in such care are in no way miracle workers. They simply help ensure that the placenta receives the cooperation it needs at the right time. Good placenta science, applied soon enough to count, will make all the difference for your pregnancy if you have complications. When it comes to testing for thrombophilia, which afflicted Shelley, much trouble can be avoided if only you're tested for thrombophilia early on. This won't necessarily happen unless you insist on it.

Even if you have other, apparently unrelated conditions, like chronic hypertension and pre-eclampsia, thrombophilia might be the main culprit. It interferes with placenta formation and quality. Research has indicated that the right anti-thrombophilia medication can cut the risk of pre-eclampsia 88% and lower the risk of abruption (where the placenta prematurely comes loose from the uterus wall) in mothers with a history of disorders including abruption, thrombophilia, chronic hypertension and pre-eclampsia.

Studies of abrupted placentas have shown severe clotting in the spiral arteries, so it makes sense to use anti-thrombotic treatment.[77] Abnormal clotting can be associated with a history or increased risk of abruption (if you've had it once, your risk of having it in a subsequent pregnancy is 20 times higher), chronic hypertension, pre-eclampsia (including high blood pressure in the mother), any serious physical injury, immune system disorders like lupus (an inflammatory disease that strikes the joints and other areas), glomerulonephritis (a kidney disease), scleroderma (a skin ailment), cocaine use (this causes severe placental vessel spasm and abruption), precipitous labor (three hours or less of labor before birth), an abnormally short umbilical cord (this can cause abruption in the final stages of labor as the baby descends in the pelvis), hydramnios (too much amniotic fluid), premature rupturing of any uterus membranes, and infection.

Abruption can be sudden or it can develop slowly, starting off as a mild condition and later turning without warning into a catastrophe. Severe abruption requires medical action at lightning speed, usually an emergency caesarean.[78] Mild abruption (depending on factors including the stage of the pregnancy) can be managed by complete bed rest in a hospital, with fetal monitoring and tests for internal bleeding or clotting.

Fetal risks from abruption include oxygen deprivation and blood loss. If the baby also has anemia (too few red blood cells or too little hemoglobin, a substance that helps move oxygen around), the risk of fetal brain damage and death increases greatly. The mother's risks from abruption include complications from emergency surgery, excessive bleeding and DIC (diffuse intravascular coagulopathy), a terrifying condition where the body's blood-clotting ability goes crazy, so that small blood vessels all over one's body become blocked by clots while at the same time any wound bleeds continuously. In severe DIC, patients bleed spontaneously from their lungs, gums, nose and any internal organ, then die.[79-81]

The best way to manage DIC is to prevent it by closely monitoring the mother's clotting processes and treating abnormality immediately. If you have any reason at all to believe you're at risk for abruption, insist on the following. Be tested for all factors related to placental thrombophilia, both genetic and acquired. (A little-known gene mutation is associated with severe placental thrombosis and related complications. Most doctors don't test for this.) Have your placental development tracked by ultrasound and Doppler from the start of the pregnancy. Be tested for chronic hypertension. (If your blood pressure doesn't drop below your pre-pregnancy levels by the 18th week, or if your blood pressure is 120/80 more than once 12 hours apart, you have hypertension issues which will likely deteriorate later in pregnancy.) Have your kidney function tested with a 24-hour urine specimen. (Checking all the urine you produce in 24 hours for protein and creatinine clearance reveals kidney health more accurately. Many women with a history of abruption or hypertension have kidney disease without knowing it. Without testing, it doesn't usually become apparent until after 20 weeks of pregnancy.)

I now come to Couvelaire uterus, a type of abruption first described by a French doctor, Alexandre Couvelaire. Here, bleeding in the uterus causes blood to be trapped under the placental center, eventually forming a blood clot big enough to push into the uterus muscle, so the uterus looks bruised. This irritates the uterus muscle, sending it into spasm. Its abnormal contractions choke the supply of blood (and oxygen) to the placenta and thus to the fetus, which dies. The contractions also exhaust the uterus muscle, leaving it paralyzed. This in turn causes more severe bleeding because normally one of the uterus muscle's functions is to control bleeding after delivery. Hysterectomy (removal of the uterus) is then the only way to save the mother from bleeding to death. This of course ends the mother's ability to have children. And with hysterectomy, too, timing is everything. In fact, this is such a drastic, life-changing step that I beg you to read and re-read the following sentences carefully:

In cases of the kind I've been describing, the decision to perform a hysterectomy can depend on whether you receive medical attention early enough for alternative action, or whether you receive it too late. If you seek attention early enough, ultrasound and other means can be used to assess your baby's condition and your own, including that of your heart and circulatory system. You can find out how much blood you've lost. (If blood is dripping down your legs, you've lost at least a pint, or half a liter. The amount of blood lost is equal to three times the volume of the clots.) Removing all blood clots from the vagina can help assess the blood loss. You can receive a blood transfusion and other fluids necessary to stabilize your condition. A large intravenous catheter will be inserted into your vein; sometimes more than one catheter must be inserted to replenish the fluids and blood you lost. Labor can be induced or an emergency caesarian can be performed if tests show that either of these steps is appropriate. If time and other circumstances allow it, steps can be taken to try to save the uterus by sealing the bleeding arteries or injecting material that can stop bleeding. Steps can be taken, if needed, to prevent atony of the uterus muscle (loss of ability to contract properly).

Speed is essential in these situations. For example, when we test for atony before it gathers full momentum, there's time to explore treatment options and make other preparations like having properly matched blood and blood components at hand. But very often the test is given too late and, by the time the atony diagnosis is confirmed, it's difficult to assemble everything needed for prompt treatment, like the right blood from the blood bank and the right medications to stimulate the uterus to contract, all of which require advance arrangement. The treatment delay can then be such that the patient can go into shock and die. Anticipation and timely preparedness are the best ways to avoid poor outcomes in both low-risk and high-risk pregnancies. Most obstetric disasters happen in pregnancies which start out being considered low-risk, and, precisely because they're considered low-risk, many justifiable anticipatory tests are skipped, allowing undetected seeds of trouble to start growing. And here's something else to think about: low-risk mothers are the largest group of pregnant women. A small fraction of them will have complications. But because there are so many low-risk mothers, the largest number of complicated pregnancies is made up of low-risk mothers, not high-risk ones as might be intuitively expected. This sounds paradoxical but it makes sense, and it's worth thinking through because it directly affects you and your baby.

Here's another odd fact. Obstetricians tend to pay more attention to women who are labeled "high risk" at the outset of their pregnancies. This is the Obstetrician's Irony. The obstetricians' good intentions make them focus on women whose high-risk pregnancies don't generate most pregnancy crises. For financial reasons, insurance companies commonly encourage the Obstetrician's Irony (although not consistently). If you fall victim to this phenomenon, you won't receive the early-pregnancy monitoring and evaluations your baby needs. Instead, care will be given not only as if all is well, but as if all will somehow continue to be well even though you and your baby have problems, which only early monitoring can detect in time to make optimal treatment possible. It's past time for the institutionalized neglect I've described here to stop and the only way you help it stop, and protect your pregnancy from it, is to speak out.

~

The problems I've just been talking about are by no means the only ones in which early screening can make a life or death difference to a pregnancy's outcome. Similar considerations apply to disorders of the placental bed, the placenta's bottom surface that touches the uterus. The bed is a common ground where your tissues intermingle with your baby's; it's where the fetus invaded your spiral arteries to tap into your blood. Anything that impacts this shared territory, or interface, impacts the whole placenta and thus the success or failure of the pregnancy. The scope for possible problems is considerable because although you share tissues with your baby in this area, your baby's needs and interests aren't always compatible with yours. This may seem strange because, after all, it's your flesh and blood. But your fetus will act to satisfy its blood supply needs regardless of your own needs. Once your unborn controls your spiral arteries, they serve not you but your baby. So if something makes you bleed fatally, you'll die before your baby does because your placental system will ensure that your last drop of blood goes not to you but to your baby. Not only will your fetus at all times absolutely control 20% of your blood, but it will also have the power to raise your blood pressure and make your heart work harder to force more blood to the placenta. This can cause conditions like preeclampsia and abruption, which can kill you. The fetus demands sustenance from a mother even when she has no more to give.

Pregnancy can therefore be thought of as a hostile symbiosis. A symbiosis is where organisms live together without mutual harm and perhaps to mutual benefit. This differs from a parasitic relationship, where an alien organism (a parasite) lives off a host to which it gives no value. A fetus isn't a parasite because it offers its mother not only immediate satisfaction of a powerful parenting urge but also a rich variety of future values including perpetuation of the mother's kind. It will, however, give priority to its own life at the expense of the mother's.

Consider the extent of that spiral artery takeover. It's generally estimated that 80 to 180 arteries are hijacked. In the context of your body, this is massive, so it's no surprise that so many pregnancy problems originate with things going wrong with spiral artery conversion. Much research has been done on this, and we now know that the presence or absence of some proteins during pregnancy's first 6 months can predict the occurrence of pre-eclampsia and other conditions. Expert use of ultrasound and Doppler technology can help us further to anticipate later problems. While prediction doesn't always translate into prevention, extensive clinical experience indicates that many complications can be prevented by paying more attention to the placental development process, especially in that critical time doctors conventionally think of as the early first trimester. Here are some conditions whose causes and contributing factors date back to the spiral artery takeover period: miscarriage in the first or second trimesters, preterm labor leading to preterm birth, preterm premature rupture of the fetal membranes, abruption, retarded fetal growth, pre-eclampsia, cerebral palsy, death of the mother and/or baby. Studies strongly show that severely flawed spiral artery conversion leads to miscarriage in the first trimester. If the flaws are serious but less severe than the flaws that cause first-trimester miscarriage, there will likely be a second-trimester crisis such as miscarriage, preterm premature rupture of the fetal membranes, fetal growth failure, pre-eclampsia or abruption.

Preterm premature rupture of the fetal membranes, also called preterm PROM, is associated with some 30% of all preterm births. Obstetricians commonly believe **PROM** is caused by infection, but the truth is that most cases result from problems with the blood vessels in the placenta or the lining of the uterus. In studies of PROM patients, up to 70% had flawed spiral artery conversion, with blood vessel damage causing ischemia (diminished blood supply), which in turn afflicts nearby tissues with inflammation that can lead to preterm labor with or without **PROM**. It's a chain reaction of causes and effects. Compelling clinical experience indicates that if blood vessel damage in the uterus originates in the lining of the uterus rather than in the placenta, **PROM** is the more likely result, while if the blood vessel damage originates in the placenta, preterm labor is likelier. The conclusion that **PROM** and preterm labor both originate in blood vessel damage is consistent with the fact that such fetuses are much likelier to have retarded growth, which we know is linked to blood vessel damage (and consequent nutrient and oxygen deprivation). PROM is also more likely in women with pre-eclampsia and abruption, both of which result from flawed spiral artery conversion and poor blood flow to the uterus.

How your body deals with blood vessel damage involves blood clotting, as we saw when I talked about thrombophilia. When blood vessels are damaged, causing loss of blood through bleeding or other blood flow abnormalities, clotting happens. A key substance in clotting is thrombin. (The medical name for a clot is "thrombus," from a Greek word meaning "lump.") Antithrombin is a substance in your blood that interferes with the clotting activity of thrombin by latching on to it to form a new substance called TAT (thrombin-antithrombin complex). When your blood is tested, the amount of TAT in it indicates whether your body is having excessive clotting. High TAT levels are associated with clotting problems including pre-eclampsia. Mothers with high TAT are likelier to experience PROM and preterm labor. (Preventing this kind of clotting problem would significantly reduce the incidence of PROM and preterm birth. Currently, eight out of 100 pregnancies experience PROM, making up 30% of premature births. Disturbingly, though preterm birth incidence varies by population and place, overall it's been rising. In 1990 in New York State eight births in 100 were preterm, but while I was preparing this book for publication it was 13, almost 62% more. Vast sums are spent annually on premature birth. The babies' hospital costs alone can be estimated by assuming an average $60,000 per baby for 450,000 babies annually, totaling $27 billion per year. This cost assumption is very conservative, being based on information from Alabama and Vermont, which I have used here because of the unavailability of reliable recent data from my home state of New York, where costs are significantly higher. This excludes the costs after preterm babies leave the hospital, which should take into account potentially lifelong care expenses for children who are disabled by prematurity. Then there's the value of the income lost by parents whose working time is shortened by caring for a disabled child. And of course the ultimate cost is the unquantifiable loss to society of the child that might have been. But when the pregnancy is closely monitored from earlier stages instead of waiting until damage is done, much fewer than one in 100 pregnancies end in **PROM**; that is, early monitoring cuts the national **PROM** average more than 90%!

This is especially sobering because this deviation from the national rate has been achieved with mothers at higher risk for preterm birth. In fact, of the mothers who are tested and treated early, 1 in 3 go into preterm labor, yet only 1 in 15 babies is delivered prematurely. The treatment is thus hugely successful, preventing 8 out of 10 preterm births. This is less than half the premature delivery rate of patients who are currently classified as low-risk. This tremendous improvement is due not to superhuman expertise or secret science but solely to scrupulous early screening, ongoing monitoring and well-established placenta science. This science recognizes that: the placenta is the key to a healthy outcome for any normal pregnancy; a damaged placenta means poor fetal growth and an impaired baby; the placenta is essentially a great blood vessel with thousands of tiny branches that nourish the fetus; the blood flow systems of both mother and fetus are very vulnerable to clotting disorders which impair the placenta, causing serious problems like preterm birth, **PROM**, pre-eclampsia, abruption, cerebral palsy, and miscarriage; clotting disorders can be treated if they're caught early enough. The successful pregnancy outcomes I've described can be obtained by examining the placenta and its blood flow every two weeks. The above information completely discredits the widespread belief that doctors and mothers can do nothing to prevent placental damage. You need to manage your pregnancy in light of the above.

None of the above means that every pregnancy should be evaluated and treated exclusively from the perspective of clotting. Any one or more of many other factors might be more important for a particular patient than clotting abnormalities. Some of those other factors might even help to counteract clotting abnormalities. Early-pregnancy screening must therefore be applied to each patient's total picture, including an examination of the mother's and father's genetics. It may seem strange to say that we make the complexity of the patient's clotting profile more manageable by putting it into the perspective of a larger complexity, but I can attest that this works; the clinical principles set out in this book make it possible to devise an effective treatment regime as early as the fifth week. Seeing the patient's clotting problems in the context of the pregnancy's larger complexity is productive because doing so recognizes each pregnancy's uniqueness. As I've noted elsewhere, no pregnancy behaves exactly the same as any other, even in the same individual. This confuses doctors who like simpler, cause-and-effect information which can be applied conveniently in replica. Complicated pregnancy, however, doesn't lend itself to this kind of simplicity. Every item of clinical information seems to insist on being related to some other item of information in the larger clinical picture. One of the ways I've sought to explain this in earlier pages, is by describing how the placenta's role as a source of precious information isn't limited to the time it spends inside your body; it continues to have invaluable information after your baby is born. Your need for clinical information doesn't end with the pregnancy, especially if you'd like to leave the door open to future pregnancies. In a laboratory, your placenta can tell us things we couldn't learn when it was inside you. Some of this information can not only be extremely useful to you in your next pregnancy effort but can even be critical to your treatment immediately after delivery. Here's an example.

We've seen how the exact location of the placenta is very important and that its best position for a successful pregnancy is in the upper part of the uterus. The strong muscles there can contract forcefully to control bleeding, whereas when the placenta lies very low in the uterus, serious bleeding problems can arise because there's less muscle there to constrict the spiral arteries when needed to control blood flow. Now, one of the things we can tell from your placenta after delivery is whether or not it was low-lying. (You'd think that routine ultrasound and other examinations would have revealed this information during the pregnancy, but this is not the case: 85% of all obstetrical ultrasounds done in the US are of questionable value because they are performed and interpreted by persons who, though professional, lack sufficient knowledge of placental physiology.) If it turns out that your placenta was low-lying, your doctor should stay with you after delivery to prevent excessive bleeding, which, unless adequate steps are taken to prevent it, could happen hours after you leave the labor room. If immediate post-delivery examination of the placenta shows that it was low-lying, such bleeding can be prevented by reaching into the vagina and pressing the lower uterus for a few minutes. This will give your body's clotting process opportunity to control the bleeding and prevent hemorrhage. But an obstetrician won't necessarily know to do this unless the placenta is examined immediately after it's expelled from the body. This and more is now illustrated by the following true story.

Chapter 16

THE DREADED WORD

I was called to a hospital recovery room bed of a young woman who'd just given birth. The resident (trainee doctor) in charge hadn't examined the placenta and so didn't realize she was on the brink of massive bleeding. She was a Jehovah's Witness whose religion forbade a blood transfusion, but, when she started bleeding and her condition destabilized, the resident ordered a transfusion. He continued to be unaware of the cause of the bleeding; the implications of a low-lying placenta didn't occur to him. The patient then refused the blood transfusion despite being told action was needed within minutes to save her life. At this point, I was brought in. I immediately saw that whatever I did had to be quick. I immediately examined the expelled placenta and could see that it had been low-lying. (This was revealed by the distance from the amniotic membrane opening from the edge of the placenta: the shorter this distance, the closer—that is, more low-lying—the placenta has been to the cervix.) Next, I swiftly examined the patient's vagina to rule out the possibility that she was bleeding from some unsuspected injury unrelated to her placental abnormality. This examination convinced me that the placenta's position was the culprit.

Gently slipping my right hand into the patient's dilated vagina, I worked it up the canal until I could feel the lower part of her uterus. At the same time, I placed my left hand on her belly so I could feel the top of her uterus through the muscle and skin. Firmly grasping this part of the uterus, I pushed it hard against my right hand, which was still inside the patient's body, braced against the lower end of the uterus. This pincer movement put pressure on the uterus from both top and bottom, constricting the blood vessels and controlling the bleeding. After about ten minutes, I removed my hand from the vagina. However, the cessation of bleeding didn't last, and as it resumed I grew tense: the patient's life was at stake. She was receiving fluids through a tube to maintain her blood volume and pressure but that wasn't going to end the problem. I inserted my right hand again, this time keeping it there until she stabilized with no longer a single drop of blood. I held this position for an hour, which exhausted me. It took so long because her considerable blood loss meant she'd also lost much of the clotting substances that control bleeding. A vicious circle, worsened by low blood pressure and the fact that diminished blood flow reduces production in the body's clotting-material factory, the liver. We almost lost this patient but all ended well and the trainee physician who'd called me in learned that the expelled placenta must always be carefully examined immediately. This emergency arose because the placenta was examined only after I arrived, when things had become much worse.

In the background of everything I've told you so far, one

dreadful word has hovered persistently: miscarriage. Other than the word "placenta", miscarriage is the common theme linking every chapter of this book. The phenomenon of miscarriage can't even begin to be understood without knowing how the placenta develops and how its developmental problems arise, while, in turn, the fact that around 75 out of 100 pregnancies don't make it can't be grasped until you understand how a nonviable fetus comes to be spontaneously lost.

A nonviable fetus is one that hasn't developed enough to survive if it's born. Viability starts appearing after week 22. By week 24, about 40 fetuses in 100 are viable. Of those born then, a small number of survivors may be able to live a relatively normal life. Most premature babies seem to have growth problems, but some catch up to a degree that can help them survive. A baby lost after 22 weeks isn't called a miscarriage but a stillbirth (if born dead) or a neonatal loss (if it's born alive and then dies). It seems unfeeling to use clinical words to talk about so terrible a thing as the loss of a baby. Medical experiences are filled with vast meaning and life-defining emotional weight, but we need the intellectual precision of scientific terms. Also, if doctors couldn't detach and distance their professional selves from the emotional content of their work, they might often become so overcome by feeling as to be rendered powerless to help their patients. So please bear with me as I explain the clinical facts of two kinds of miscarriage: sporadic and recurrent. Sporadic (occasional) miscarriages don't necessarily indicate a major problem with the mother's ability to have children. Recurrent (frequently repeating) miscarriages, however, can mean trouble of this kind, and here again I have expressed my criticism of prevailing obstetric habits and attitudes. I won't say most obstetricians ignore sporadic miscarriages, but

I believe most obstetricians tend not to be very concerned about them, seeing them as isolated accidents. And they often are. Many women with sporadic miscarriages go on to have normal pregnancies without further losses. Most doctors recommend no special tests or treatment for a woman whose first pregnancy miscarries. Most sporadic miscarriages result from flawed chromosomes or random womb events that damage the embryo or placenta. (A chromosome is a bundle of genes, remember, a gene being a packet of chemical instructions inherited from our parents, spelling out our developmental programming.) Some 40% to 60% of first miscarriages have been reported to be genetically abnormal.

With more than one miscarriage, however, genetic abnormality tends to feature less with each loss. In recurrent miscarriage, just seven in 100 losses involve chromosome defects (i.e., 93% of recurrent miscarriages are caused not by genetic problems, which are generally beyond our present powers of correction, but by relatively much simpler accidents in the uterus). And most can probably be prevented if we identify the cause early enough to correct it. We can't yet fix the chromosome defects that cause the other 7% of losses, though. Most such defects are lethal and the embryo never makes it to viability. The most common chromosomal defect that's compatible with life in about 80% of cases is Down syndrome. With prenatal diagnosis of lethal chromosomal defects, the patient can either end the pregnancy and try again or allow it to proceed. If it's left to proceed the embryo either dies or is born severely impaired. Of babies diagnosed with the rare trisomy 18, or Edward's syndrome, only 20% are born alive, and they are severely impaired physically and mentally. Most die in five years. The oldest known survivor made it to some 15 years. Only a few parents allow such pregnancies to continue.

I've had two such cases which changed my idea of what is normal. Doctors are trained to look at things objectively, through the lens of measurable evidence, but this comes at a cost of often missing the implications of human feelings, values and other non-material aspects of life. In the two cases I've just mentioned, both babies died, but their parents demanded and received full care for them while this was possible. One insisted on treatment for diabetes with daily insulin injections for both mother and baby. The first baby died on the third day of life, the day after open-heart surgery for a major cardiac defect. The second died minutes before birth. Both mothers insisted on giving their babies every chance that any other baby would get. I have never seen any bereaved person so much at peace as these mothers. They felt their babies would be with them forever even though they'd been unable to stay.

For decades, recurrent miscarriage has been diagnosed after three losses each occurring in the first 24 weeks. This definition began when it was far harder than it is today either to tell why a pregnancy failed or to do much to prevent a fourth miscarriage. Patients with three losses were essentially labeled as recurrent losers. This stereotype continues today (i.e., obstetricians are still diagnosing with obsolete criteria that date back more than half a century). This is all the more distressing because, as I've discussed earlier, way back then most women started raising families at an early age and devoted much of their lives to it, while women today commonly pursue careers first, starting a family only in their 30s and allocating fewer years to having children, which they then do at a time of life when they face a higher risk of placental and other physiological problems. Most pregnant women today are over 30. In the last 45 years or so, the age of women having their first child has risen hugely. According to a report by an authoritative international body, the Organization for Economic Co-operation and Development (OECD), in most developed countries, the median age of first-time mothers is between around 30 and 32. However, the United States contains more population variety than many other developed countries and some parts of the US contain so many poor people that those areas resemble underdeveloped rather than developed countries. No surprise then that some 80% of first pregnancies in the US in 2012 were in mothers older than 25. But the first-time age figure rises as you look at more educated and more financially well-off US communities. The average age of the main clinical databank of this book (drawn from mothers in the New York area) is around 38. Many are in their fifties! Women wanting babies after 35 face heightened risks of many disorders including diabetes, hypertension and illnesses of the heart, blood vessels (including clotting) and thyroid.

So don't be satisfied with the prevailing antiquated attitude to recurrent miscarriage. If you lose a baby, let your doctor know in no uncertain terms that you're not prepared to have it shrugged off as an accident of nature. Insist that you'll regard it as a serious medical oversight if every effort isn't made to investigate the reasons for a loss, including a first-time one. Such an investigation is in your interest at any age but especially after 35. Any woman who loses her first pregnancy after 35 can become infertile if the cause isn't diagnosed and treated immediately. After 35, your ovarian function can decline very quickly. The clock is ticking. You can't afford to try three times before an investigation is done.

You also need to know that, in addition to using an outdated prevailing diagnostic approach, many doctors tend to pigeonhole patients into groups and deal with them according to guidelines for

THE DREADED WORD

that group instead of seeing each patient as a unique individual. A woman of 38 can spend a fortune on medical help to get pregnant and then, after pregnancy failure, find herself placed in the same general patient category as a first-timer of 22 who's conceived naturally. This doesn't make sense. Again, no individual doctor deserves blame for this foolish and dangerous situation. Doctors are now given guidelines as part of the way their profession is run, including pressure from insurance companies. In addition to helping less competent doctors do their jobs, a major aim of the guidelines is to reduce costs. This looks good when the focus is on numbers rather than on people. Medically, it plays out less well. For example, studies indicate that about 2 in 100 normal fetuses die after 22 weeks, while in complicated pregnancies up to 20 in 100 die, depending on the kind of complication. But the guidelines don't focus on this 20% death rate.[82] They focus on the 80 out of 100 babies that survive. In accounting-based medicine, where cost-and-profit analysis is the highest priority, the medical administration system considers a 20% death rate acceptable! It's hard for me to write about this without becoming very angry, and my guess is it will make you angry too. A 20% death rate acceptable? The mother whose baby is among the "acceptable losses" isn't losing 20% of anything. She's losing 100% of her baby and possibly of her chances of ever having a child. Aside from the inherent wrongness of allowing that to happen, and the loss to society of the person her baby might have become, such an event can impair that woman with lifelong illnesses including severe depression. But this cost too isn't recognized by profit-based medicine. It's estimated that half a million babies a year die in recurrent miscarriage, with 7% being genetically abnormal. The rest (465,000 babies) can potentially be saved and only about 6%

are lost due to problems medical science can't figure out. The explainable deaths are most frequently attributed to infections, clotting problems (in at least 60% of cases), problems with the formation of the mother's body (e.g., her uterus and cervix), defects in the fetus's chromosomes or in the formation of its body (these last two problems overlap because most chromosome defects cause or contribute to flawed body development), and hormone abnormalities.[1, 83]

Let's briefly look at these problems. First: infection is often wrongly blamed for recurrent miscarriage. Clinical evidence indicates infections aren't a significant cause of recurrent miscarriage or preterm birth. An infection can't easily hide undetected in your genital tract. Only patients with symptoms should be tested for infections; routinely testing recurrent-miscarriage patients isn't sensible. The misguided focus on infection as a significant cause of recurrent miscarriage is largely due to the inflammation that's commonly caused by tissue damage in the placenta and surrounding areas in most pregnancy losses. There are two kinds of inflammation, infectious and non-infectious, and we must distinguish between them. Considerable clinical evidence associates pregnancy complications less with infectious than non-infectious inflammation. Inflammation can trigger abnormal clotting in placental blood vessels, and we've seen that the placenta is in effect a huge blood vessel with lots of tiny branches. We've also seen that blood vessel events, including clotting, is connected with many pregnancy issues. Recurrent miscarriage is no exception.

I've talked about immune system disorders. In one of these, APS (antiphospholipid antibody syndrome), your immune system mistakenly starts making antibodies that hunt down your phospholipids, essential fats which occur everywhere. This spree by

THE DREADED WORD

crazed antibodies damages blood vessels, which triggers clotting. APS and things connected with it can cause serious problems at various stages of pregnancy. They can interfere with implantation and spiral artery conversion; they can cause placental clotting and poor placental development, conditions which underlie most pregnancy complications like growth restriction, pre-eclampsia, preterm birth, abruption and fetal death. Mothers with APS have an 80% chance of miscarriage ... but the clinical methods described in this book can cut this risk to just 2% IF they're applied from the earliest stages of pregnancy. The miscarriage triggers that arise from immune system problems include rogue behavior by the Natural Killer (NK) cells which, as we've seen, are particularly fierce attack dogs whose job is to defend your body by killing anything they perceive as foreign. Although your embryo is partly foreign because of the paternal half of its genes, a healthy immune system will exempt it from attack by the NK cells; but this exemption can fail. The NK cell attack on the fetal tissues can then stop you from falling pregnant at all, and if you do conceive you might experience multiple miscarriages, or complications involving placental malformation. If these problems are caught early enough, they can be fixed with substances that restore the immune system's control of the NK cells.

NK cell abnormality tends to be absent from common medical explanations of recurrent miscarriage. This is because history is repeating itself. APS and its related clotting issues are today among the most common explanations of recurrent miscarriage, but many doctors dismissed them for decades before finally acknowledging their role. Similarly, many doctors today refuse to recognize the link between NK cell abnormality and recurrent miscarriage even though it's been validated by extensive clinical observation. I'm sure this too will change, but the slowness of recognition is meanwhile arguably costing the lives of many babies who could be saved, and preventing many mothers from having babies sooner, if at all. It's poignant and chilling to think of all the damage and suffering being needlessly inflicted by this failure of our medical establishment.

Regarding the connection between recurrent miscarriage and maternal anatomical problems (e.g., with the uterus and/or cervix), the worst anatomical problem is uterus didelphys, where the uterus develops into two separate organs, each half normal size, with two of everything, sometimes even two separate vaginal cavities. Less severe is a bicornuate uterus, with one cervix (opening) but two internal cavities. The least severe is a uterine septum, with one cervix and one internal cavity, but the cavity is divided by a wall (septum). This can cause impaired growth, prematurity and miscarriage. Neither of the first two abnormalities can be fixed; doctors must just do their best to help the baby cope and grow as best as possible. But a uterine septum can be removed with surgery via hysteroscopy, which increases the odds of a successful pregnancy outcome. Any expert should be able to perform such a procedure. However, substantial clinical evidence indicates that these uterine defects don't cause recurrent miscarriage as much as many doctors think, nor do they usually cause first-trimester loss. I've found that mothers with these issues have increased risk of preterm labor (generally around week 22), but that recurrent pregnancy loss is rarely associated with anatomical uterine abnormalities. It's thus very disturbing that most of these women's miscarriages are often too easily blamed on their anatomical problem without investigation of other possible causes. A compelling mass of clinical observations over many years indicates that anatomical-defect patients seeking specialized care after recurrent pregnancy loss overwhelmingly tend to have uninvestigated clotting disorders. This again illustrates the medical establishment's blind spot regarding the early-stage placental origins of many pregnancy problems, a widespread, almost perverse desire to look anywhere except at that area which is the foundation of successful pregnancies and the problems that bedevil them. This same situation applies to fibroids, benign uterine growths which rarely cause pregnancy loss yet are often blamed for it. Because fibroids occur in some 30% of women of child-bearing age, blaming them is easier than looking further. But my files contain no case where fibroids caused a baby to be lost to a mother who was treated properly and in good time for any clotting disorder. Evidence suggests fibroids can't threaten a pregnancy until the second trimester, and then only if the placenta is attached to a large fibroid (this increases abruption risk). I have case histories of many patients with fibroids but not one includes such complications. Medical textbooks describe fibroids as a serious contributor to miscarriage, but I've found this to be at best only partly true; fibroids can cause infertility or pregnancy loss if and when they disturb the uterus cavity or block the fallopian tubes by compression. In such cases, myomectomy (surgical removal of fibroids) can be done. The type of surgery will depend on factors including the fibroids' location, number and size. Myomectomy can scar the uterus enough to preclude future natural childbirth afterwards for fear of uterine rupture, so if you've had a myomectomy, ask your doctor if natural birth is safe for you or if a caesarean section is necessary.

Chapter 17

THE WOMB AS A BLOOD-CLOT BOMB

Our discussion of commonly attributed causes of recurrent miscarriage now brings us to genetic defects, including fetal anatomy problems resulting from chromosome problems. Given that we need 46 chromosomes (23 from each parent), any deviation from this number or their healthy arrangement is a problem, with different chromosome abnormalities causing different problems, from miscarriage in the first 12 weeks to Down syndrome or molar pregnancy, where the placenta grows with no fetus, a condition that must be caught and treated soon to avoid lethal cancer. Genes, then, are undeniably important in pregnancy. Yet genetic disorders too can easily be used as an excuse not to spend time looking at other causes of recurrent miscarriage, and to bypass massive evidence that by far the most common cause for recurrent miscarriage is some form of complex clotting disorder.

Sometimes, of course, such a disorder can include a genetic problem. For example, there's a genetic mutation that reduces the body's ability to dissolve clots. Such problems can depend on your ethnicity. African-American women are more likely than Caucasian women to have immune system clotting disorders, but less likely to have genetic clotting disorders. But the most important point is that, while some genetic defects can be catastrophic, genetic influence most often tends to be just one aspect among a large array of influences that potentially determine whether or not you'll lose a baby, and, if a loss is coming, when. My clinical files compellingly indicate that if we want to name any problem area that looms largest as a contributor to recurrent miscarriage, it's placenta-related clotting problems, plural because this isn't a single neatly identifiable problem but a cluster of problems, each with multiple contributing factors working together in a highly individual way from pregnancy to pregnancy. Each case is unique, requiring individual early-pregnancy testing rather than generic classification and interpretation in terms of guidelines which framed for groups rather than individual women and individual babies. The complex, multi-factorial and highly individual nature of miscarriage is further underlined by what doctors call "unexplained miscarriage," which, as I've said elsewhere, simply means they have failed to identify the cause. Of course, even when doctors do everything they can to investigate, the cause may still elude them. Doctors aren't superhuman. The immensity of nature is always infinitely greater than our knowledge. However, we know enough about miscarriages to say confidently that our ignorance of nature is too often invoked as a handy excuse. In today's medical world, "unexplained miscarriage" is usually a cop-out. My clinical files, encompassing decades of cases, reference very few unexplained miscarriages if any. There are miscarriages whose specific character is harder than others to isolate, but generally, a group of highly likely causes rewards adequate investigation, suggesting that an "unexplained" miscarriage simply tends to be an insufficiently investigated one, or one where the doctor isn't familiar enough with the range of possible causes and their intricate potential connections (e.g., the link that can exist between genes and clotting). Although, as I've said, genes can also be abused as a catch-all excuse for everything we can't understand, but this doesn't mean they aren't very important. They're the language in which the story of our bodies is written, and, as we evolve as a species, this story changes in ways that aren't always in our best interests, as is illustrated by the "thrifty gene" theory. Scientists who support this theory believe some people get fat more easily than others because of a type of gene that's outlived its usefulness. According to them, our ancestors developed genes to store energy in the form of body fat so they could use this stored energy when food became scarce. People with these genes were more likely to survive during periods of prolonged winters and thus more likely to pass their genes to next generations. In contrast, people without the thrifty gene were more likely to die from harsh winters when food supplies were scarce and their fat deposits limited. Their shorter lives limited their offspring and thus the transmission of their genes to the next generation. But supposedly, these same genes which once helped us are now in a sense our enemy, because today we have much more food than our ancestors did, so the ease with which we take on fat (with the help of these genes) is causing widespread obesity, which is dangerous to our health.

    It's not unreasonable to imagine that similar considerations might apply to our bodies' ability to clot blood. Our cave-dwelling ancestors faced more physical dangers than we do (like being attacked by wild animals), so they were at higher risk of bleeding to death. As there were no high-tech pregnancy clinics in those early times, many women bled to death in childbirth. The survivors were the ones whose genes improved their clotting ability. And because they transmitted these genes to their children, each generation's clotting ability steadily became stronger. These suppositions suggest that after thousands of years we now have an inbuilt tendency to easy clotting. Modern lifestyles and health care, however, make this both unnecessary and potentially dangerous, increasing our risk of heart attacks, strokes and pregnancy complications. The rise in mothers' ages makes matters worse. Just being pregnant in itself increases a woman's proneness to clotting, and clotting problems worsen with age. Put together these facts mean a pregnant woman is a clotting bomb ticking away ominously. We now know enough to defuse the bomb but only if we act early enough and recognize the placenta's role at the center of this situation as the mother-baby blood-vessel link, in which clotting problems can cause poor placental development leading to complications including preterm birth, fetal growth failure, fetal death and pre-eclampsia, with improper placental formation being the main cause of recurrent first-trimester miscarriages. And while miscarriage in the first 22 weeks is horrific, it's no less awful at 35 weeks, or to have a brain-damaged baby. Early screening is essential, not only to detect and treat clotting problems that can contribute to such disasters, but also to check for chromosome defects, especially as women over 35 have such a higher chance of having a Down syndrome baby.

Down syndrome itself illustrates how closely the many factors affecting pregnancy are connected. In the 1980s, the risk of Down syndrome and some other abnormalities was found to be higher in mothers with low levels of a substance called maternal serum alpha-fetoprotein or MS-AFP, while the risk of spina bifida or other anatomical defects was higher if the MS-AFP was unusually high. A few years later, it became clear from several scientific studies that, even if they were carrying genetically normal babies, women with high MS-AFP levels were at higher risk for severe placenta-related complications and poor outcomes including preterm PROM, severe growth failure, abruption, pre-eclampsia and for the baby's death before or at birth. These high-MS-AFP patients were labeled as high-risk, but nothing was done to prevent the bad outcomes.[84-87]

I was then working at a major research institution where I saw thousands of patients a year. What I saw made it clear to me that the placentas of high-MS-AFP patients differed significantly from those of women with normal MS-AFP. The high-MS-AFP mothers had more (and bigger) placental lakes. A placental lake is a pool of blood in the placenta or on its surface. On ultrasound screens, these phenomena appeared as black patches which, at that time, were thought to be unproblematic, open intervillous spaces. But as ultrasound technology improved, we could see they were places without villi and that they contained maternal blood, which in some patients was clotted. I suspected clotting of fetal or maternal blood had created these areas, damaging the villi, with this damage allowing fetal AFP (alpha-fetoprotein) to enter the mother's bloodstream and raise her MS-AFP. And it dawned on me that the placental damage was the cause of the poor outcomes of these pregnancies.

Many investigators in those days thought most problems start in the mother's circulation, not the fetus's. But fetal clotting (fetal thrombotic vasculopathy or FTV) is a big problem, damaging fetal blood vessel walls and making the otherwise selective placental membrane let fetal AFP into the mother's blood. This damage usually involves thrombosis and increasingly destroys placental tissue until the whole placenta fails. And placental failure is a road to all pregnancy complications, including the problems of patients with "unexplained" MS-AFP elevation. As my co-workers and I advanced our understanding of this (and as ultrasound technology improved) and we treated patients more knowledgeably with anticoagulants, pregnancy outcomes got better. Further, with time, tests became available to identify many aspects of clotting abnormalities associated with placental thrombosis. However, despite years of evidence about the clotting basis of "unexplained" MS-AFP elevation, most childbirth doctors still ignore these findings and leave such patients untreated. Today's obstetric students usually aren't taught much, if anything, about "unexplained" MS-AFP.

One reason for this is the way new information gets documented. Once, AFP was the only substance measured when a mother's blood was tested for spina bifida and Down syndrome. Today, doctors test for four substances. When the results come back, the AFP component tends to be overshadowed by the other three results and it's thus mostly ignored. If the other results are OK, an elevated AFP result is often not even discussed. These circumstances can lead to the untreated development of a pregnancy complication, which could be serious enough to make the mother lose her baby. We now know that the presence of two substances called **PAPP-A** (pregnancy associated plasma protein) and beta-hCG (the beta chain of chorionic gonadotropin) can indicate conditions like Down syndrome. A high PAPP-A result is good. A low result means increased risk for Down syndrome.

All this is, again, crucially connected with your placenta. A few years after doctors starting using the PAPP-A test, it was noticed that an abnormally low PAPP-A result (even in a genetically normal baby) is associated with complications and poor pregnancy outcomes, with the risk of the baby's death becoming several times greater. The medical profession has responded to this important finding by continuing to manage such patients in the same way as other high-risk patients are conventionally managed, with frequent ultrasound evaluations and check-ups in the last trimester. This management hasn't succeeded in improving the pregnancy success rate. Mothers with abnormally low PAPP-A still experience severe complications even if they're monitored more frequently than patients with normal PAPP-A. Why? Because most physicians still don't make the connection between a low PAPP-A result and an unhealthy placenta. If a doctor tests a mother but doesn't treat the placenta after seeing a low PAPP-A result, what is the point of having this placental information? This situation exists because of the poor understanding of the placenta that prevails in today's medical world.

A recent study found that monitoring alone made no difference to the complications of mothers with low PAPP-A and a small placenta; even with ultrasound monitoring every two weeks, 17% of these babies died before birth and 3% died after birth, a dreadful and wholly unacceptable statistic. Even scarier is that the investigators who conducted this study made absolutely no recommendations about how to improve the situation. They, too, were apparently unaware of the need to treat the placenta! It's clear that the scientific community is confused about the placenta. All the major published studies tend to report findings about placental dysfunction without making any apparent effort to explain the causes.[88-92]

In short, the above information boils down to this picture of events: the villi tissues (the villi being the "fingers" of tissue inside the intervillous space, which is bathed in maternal blood) produce PAPP-A; if PAPP-A is low, the tissue cells aren't well, which could mean the placenta won't be able to supply the baby with enough food and oxygen; this picture, supported by extensive evidence, explains a lot by making a minimum of assumptions, and it can be tested in experiments. But experiments on people would face ethical and legal barriers because they'd require a willingness to let some mothers and/or babies be harmed or even die to prove a point, while experiments with animals wouldn't give us conclusive results as the placentas of various species differ too much. Also, an appropriate placental study of animals would cost so much it would be difficult to fund it. This means we must work with the evidence we have, which is solid, being based on extensive clinical experience which shows compellingly that low PAPP-A is connected to placental problems that lead to poor pregnancy outcomes. The more doctors act on this mass of available evidence, the more evidence we'll get.

We know the placenta is abnormally small in mothers with low PAPP-A. We know that relatively normal placentas are associated with fewer complications than abnormally small ones. This knowledge powerfully indicates that complications in low PAPP-A pregnancies arise from the link between low PAPP-A and physical damage of placental tissue. It will help you understand this further if you compare the problems of high AFP and low PAPP-A. The placenta doesn't produce AFP. A high amount of AFP in maternal blood is caused by AFP leaking from the baby's blood to the mother's blood through a damaged placental membrane. But low PAPP-A is different. This is produced by the placenta tissue. But the AFP and PAPP-A problems have this in common: both have to do with whether the placenta structure is healthy. In pregnancies with high AFP and placental damage from clotting, poor outcomes are directly related to the degree of placental damage; the worse the damage, the more AFP appears in the mother's blood. Likewise, in pregnancies with low PAPP-A and placental damage, placental size correlates directly with PAPP-A levels. In some patients with low PAPP-A, the placental size might be normal, but the placenta function is reduced. This stands to reason. As the placenta is the baby's only food supplier any reduction in its size or its function will lead to problems like growth failure, preterm premature rupture of membranes, preeclampsia, fetal death, preterm birth and newborn death.

Despite the mass of evidence suggesting that, if we stop or correct the damage to the placenta, we could reduce or even end these tragic occurrences, there are no published studies of this except for those my clinical team and I have produced, drawing on data amassed over decades dating back to the days before tests became available to diagnose clotting disorders. Every year I see a distressing number of patients whose abnormal PAPP-A and/or MS-AFP are ignored by their doctors, imperiling the baby's life. While I was seeing this book to publication, a patient lost her baby before my eyes because of this ignorance. Had this patient been sent to me just two weeks earlier, she would have had a premature but healthy baby. Had I seen her immediately after the abnormal test result (i.e., four weeks before, she would have had a healthy full- term pregnancy). Our studies indicate that treatment with blood thinners normalizes the outcomes of patients with low PAPP-A and that potential placental clotting problems must be investigated from the earliest stages of the pregnancy. Our anticoagulation treatment has achieved excellent results, including in cases of mothers with elevated AFP. The use of these treatments has significantly reduced complications and completely eliminated fetal death in the patients studied. Further, since clotting tests became commercially available in the 1990s, we've documented the presence of clotting disorders in patients with unexplained AFP elevation and have in recent years been doing similar work with low-PAPP-A mothers.

Many researchers recommend treating low-PAPP-A mothers as high-risk patients, but this vague advice dodges the real question: What can the obstetrician DO for such a mother? How helpful is it to call a pregnancy "high-risk" without addressing the nature of the risk? Also, applying so vague a label can make the mother so anxious that her stress becomes a risk factor on its own. This is a major reason why you need to educate yourself about pregnancy risks. Ultimately you, not your doctor, are responsible for yourself and your baby. As I hope I've already made clear, I don't want to undermine your trust in your doctor, which is a cornerstone of your medical care. But this relationship works best as a collaboration, given that physicians are constrained not only by the boundaries of human knowledge but also by trends of attitude, just as fashions come and go in other fields. Consider that doctors once gave patients advice that no doctor would subscribe today. They did so not because they were unethical or inept, but because that advice was conventional medical establishment practice at the time, and, when I speak of doctors, I'm not speaking about individual ones; I'm referring to the conventional practices of today's medical establishment, which includes powerful insurance companies. However, your own contact with the medical establishment is via your own doctor, so while you shouldn't take your frustrations with the medical establishment out on your doctor, you should tell your doctor how you want your pregnancy managed, contrary to the common perception of patients as passive recipients of a doctor's decisions. Listen to your doctor respectfully, then contribute your views and requirements. It's your body. A poor understanding of the placenta is rampant in the medical profession, so do assert your and your baby's rights.

You may hear opposition to using a treatment that's not backed by large-scale clinical studies, yet many doctors use treatments whose supposed benefits aren't supported by evidence. Medical practice is an applied profession that not only uses evidence from large-scale clinical studies but also relies heavily, even perhaps mainly, on what's found to work in clinical experience. But many doctors have a double standard about this, selectively citing the authority of clinical experience to justify practices they've grown used to while rejecting this same authority when it's cited on behalf of a new practice requiring them to change their ways. The reason: simply habit. A classic example is the use of two substances used to treat preterm labor: magnesium sulfate and terbutaline. They don't just lack benefit; there is compelling evidence that they can harm both mother and baby. Yet long after this evidence became available, they continued to be used by obstetricians who were accustomed to them and were unwilling to switch to new medications whose safety had been scientifically validated. This reflects a serious problem that's pervasive in medicine: the herd mentality. Members of a herd feel comfortable to follow the herd even when it's going in a dangerous direction. Doctors use the phrase "standard of care" to mean the most commonly accepted way of handling a medical situation. It sounds good. "Standard" and "care" are reassuring words. But the standard care is open to the criticism that it often represents nothing more than herd mentality: i.e., it's a standard not because it has medical merit, but just because a lot of doctors like it, and they like it for no other reason than they're used to it.[93-98]

Consider the standard of care for pregnancy complications associated with low PAPP-A. Much evidence indicates that these are caused by placental deficiencies which can be corrected, but, because this evidence is derived from clinical experience, the standard of care for placental weaknesses associated with low PAPP-A is to do nothing and allow these problems to take their course without treatment. This is perfectly acceptable among obstetricians, most of whom nod their heads in comfortable agreement that nothing can be done, in defiance of clear and compelling evidence to the contrary. Eventually, the tide turns in these situations, and new treatments are eventually accepted. Sometimes this will happen only after decades, while, meanwhile, physicians who stand up to the inertia can suffer ridicule even when their results are successful. I speak from experience.

In 1987, I was one of the few doctors who started using transvaginal ultrasound for cervical and preterm labor problems. In ordinary sonograms, an imaging instrument is placed on the abdomen; in transvaginal ultrasound, it's gently placed in the vagina, generally obtaining far better womb imagery. This went against familiar custom and the obstetric profession reacted angrily. I was mocked. There were hints that I didn't have patient interests at heart and was just after more money (although at that time I didn't charge my patients for such screening). But my clinical team and I knew we had facts, sound sense and good results on our side: along with other doctors committed to the new approach, we continued with transvaginal ultrasound despite the sneers. After 15 years or so, it started entering into general use, and today it's part of the "standard of care." Similar medical shunning has bedeviled the introduction, by myself and other breakaway doctors, of other approaches beyond our profession's zone of habits, like the use of certain anti-clotting medications for thrombophilia and other clotting disorders and of Doppler ultrasound to measure fetal blood flow and vascular resistance. (As I've explained elsewhere, this technology uses sound to track the movement of blood cells.) The still ongoing struggle to get more doctors to use Doppler illustrates how hard it can be to introduce life-saving innovations. Several of the US's major health insurance companies argue that Doppler technology is "experimental" despite its decades-long, established clinical application, and use this as an excuse not to pay for its inclusion in patient care. I consider this to be an unconscionable evasion of the medical care responsibilities that these companies owe their paying members. (Other insurers have come to allow limited coverage of its inclusion.) This clever verbal maneuvering on the part of the insurers, in order to further inflate their wallets, comes at the expense of the health of their members, and their members' babies. It also comes at the cost of doctors who find themselves ethically compelled, from time to time, to make up for the insurers' exclusion of Doppler services by undertaking supplementary studies for some patients even when they know they will not receive payment for these studies. I myself have provided such unpaid-for supplementary studies of multiple blood vessels in multiple patient visits without the benefit of insurance-covered Doppler, in order to gain a necessarily complete picture of the health of these patients and their babies. This inefficiently burdens physicians and ultimately hurts the resources of the healthcare system, rendering ill service to mothers and babies, and it is brought about solely by the insurers' greed. Doppler's ability to save fetal lives has been clearly shown, but its use calls for the painstaking acquisition of special knowledge of the heart and blood vessel physiology of fetus and mothers, at a level that very few obstetricians command.[99-102] By contrast, the more popular alternative to Doppler involves the comparatively simple use of a machine to measure the fetal heart rate. This method is called a non-stress test (NST), certainly a reassuring name. Who wants stress? It's a misleading name, though. It seems to imply the leading alternative, Doppler imaging, does inflict stress on the mother or fetus, which isn't true. Most problematic of all is that there's no proof whatsoever that an NST can protect fetuses from serious complications, including some fatal ones.[103-106] Yet NST is the standard of care while fetal and uteroplacental Doppler is rarely used. As a result, hundreds of thousands of babies suffer short-term and long-term health problems, and many die. Tragically, this is how our medical system works. Doctors must often be willing to risk ridicule to innovate, because innovation means challenging convenient convention.

There are, then, more medical approaches available to you and your unborn baby than you'll necessarily hear about unless you proactively seek them out. Quiz your doctor about alternative treatments. Insist on knowing all the options open to you, not only those within the prevailing standard of care. Let your doctor know you're aware that Doppler ultrasound is safe for fetuses and mothers, and that there's a proven link between placental thrombosis and fetal complications similar to those in patients with high AFP and/or low PAPP-A, so, if you have high AFP, or low PAPP-A this mustn't be ignored even if you and your fetus seem healthy enough otherwise. High AFP or low PAPP-A can be life-determining warning signals. Low PAPP-A isn't a problem per se; its association with damaged and/or small placentas means we must see it as the smoke from the hidden fire of damaged villi and placental thrombosis; the more damaged villi, the higher your chance of pregnancy complications. Clinical experience has revealed that most, if not all, patients with low PAPP-A did just as well as patients without low PAPP-A, provided all were treated with anti-clotting medication.

Before coming in for examination and treatment according to the placenta-based pregnancy care philosophy I've been describing to you, most of these patients had suffered complications relating to placental failure. All had clotting problems. They were treated successfully with low-molecular-weight heparin and aspirin. Repeated successes with low PAPP-A patients shows their problems can be treated very effectively with anti-clotting medication and that they can achieve healthy, full-term pregnancies.[107, 108] My clinical colleagues and I have published this information in peer-reviewed medical journals but, given the medical establishment's ponderous slowness, don't hold your breath waiting for these placenta-based methods to become the standard of care.

Tell your doctor you know lives have been saved by giving anti-clotting medication to patients with unexplained high AFP; that conditions causing clotting disorders (thrombophilia) lead to clotting in the placenta, which in turn leads to bad pregnancy outcomes; that anti-clotting treatment during pregnancy is safe and reduces bad pregnancy outcomes; and that all this knowledge must be used to formulate the right treatment for you as an individual, even if it means breaking away from the comfortable, conventional, collectively formulated standard of care.[109]

All this sounds, I realize, like an uphill battle against entrenched medical habits, but the good news is that this information can benefit you and your baby now, without waiting for the medical profession to catch up. To drive home the point that even tiny bits of information can make a profound difference to your pregnancy, let me tell you the story of the patient I'll call Fran.

Chapter 18

FRAN'S STORY

Fran discovered that a mother seeking the truth behind a series of miscarriages can be like a sleuth solving a murder mystery: the secret may lie in just one apparently small, overlooked clue.

Time and time again, Fran miscarried. For four frustrating, depressing years, she and her husband Bernard tried to sustain a pregnancy. With the dedication of a scholar trying to crack the code of a baffling ancient language, they searched relentlessly to learn why she was repeatedly miscarrying. They consulted experts. A reproductive endocrinologist said she just had "bad eggs." Another specialist said she had "blocked tubes." Another blamed her age. (She was in her 30s.) And she would later recall that not one of these authorities treated her for any specific pregnancy-related problem, or diagnosed any such problem, or even tested her blood. Her miscarriages were just accepted as a feature of who she was, as if she was destined not to have a baby.

After deciding to try her first in vitro fertilization (IVF), she also decided to see one more specialist as a last resort. What could she lose? By then she was 36. The doctor she chose happened to be me. The first thing I did was to send her for extensive blood tests. These showed she had a clotting disease, genetic thrombophilia, that can be successfully treated with anticoagulants and aspirin. She also had two immune system disorders. But there was a deeper problem which wasn't going to show itself so easily.

With IVF she conceived, her thrombophilia treatment was having apparently good results, and she was being monitored with ultrasound every two weeks with no problems showing up. Then, suddenly, at 16 weeks a scan showed that Fran's chorion, the protective membrane around the baby, had severely damaged villi, those finger-shaped projections that stick out from the chorion and infuse fresh food and oxygen into the baby's bloodstream. This wasn't only unexpected but inconsistent with her known medical history and treatment. Her immune system disorders weren't associated with these problems. On the assumption that her thrombophilia might somehow have caused the damage despite her treatment for it, which had seemed to be working, Fran's anticoagulant dose was doubled. If the thrombophilia was the culprit, the problem could now be expected to end. However, two more weeks passed and not only was there no recovery, but the villi damage worsened. Something other than thrombophilia was affecting Fran's placenta. But what?

A new bout of blood testing showed a new immune system problem. Fran had abnormally aggressive NK (natural killer) cells, which as we've seen are a part of your immune system that can go rogue, mistakenly attacking things they shouldn't. Much about these cells is still mysterious. Some experts have speculated that rogue NK activity might play roles in disorders including multiple sclerosis and diabetes. In pregnancy, we know crazed NK cells can target the chorionic villi and the baby's own blood vessels. This, we found, was happening to Fran.

Her confused immune system was attacking not only her own tissues but the baby's too. Now, anticoagulant medication, which counteracts the clotting caused by thrombophilia, can also mildly dampen the body's immune system. In Fran's case, this benign side effect had helped to slow down the onset of her NK cell problem. But while this was good, it had also unfortunately masked the NK problem, which consequently went unnoticed and thus untreated until it became too aggressive to escape detection.

Fran was treated with daily steroids and fortnightly lipid (fat) emulsion injections, which can usually combat immune system disorders, although in this case this tried and tested method couldn't cope: there were too many wild NK cells and their activity had grown too vigorous under the cloak of stealth, which, ironically, had been provided by Fran's otherwise protective anticoagulant medications. The NK army overwhelmed her physiological system, and at 22 weeks she lost the baby. Beyond being a catastrophe for Fran and Bernard, I myself was profoundly affected by the loss. Despite the aloof professional detachment that doctors are supposed to observe, doctors can take it very personally when things go badly for a patient. Aside from human solidarity and sympathy, doctors, being only human, can feel a blow to their sense of worth when disaster befalls a patient who has looked to the physician's skill for protection. The doctor can then hold a kind of grudge against the sickness and this never burns so fiercely as in the face of the loss of a life which hasn't yet even had a chance to begin; this feels like the ultimate rebuff of the doctor's sacred mission to serve life. The self-protective psychology of many doctors protects them against pregnancy loss by making them appear, to themselves and others, to be capable of shrugging it off, but other doctors react to the loss of a life on their watch with a deep, almost obsessive desire to do whatever they can to see that such disasters stop happening, on the basis that, if we can't bring back a departed life, then at least we can wage a more fiery war against the enemy that took the life. I confess to belonging to this category, and this signifies no pretension to superiority over my more dispassionate colleagues; it is just a fact of difference in personality and philosophy. In Fran's case, I had no doubt that I would feel a bit better if I could find out why this had happened. While I had been doing this work long enough to understand the overall mechanics of the NK cells' behavior, my intuition told me there was more to the story than met the eye. And my interest was not just academic but also fundamentally practical, because Fran still wanted a child. If the cause of her latest loss could be found, might that not help her break down the wall that some unknown physiological process had erected between her and her desire for motherhood?

I sent a sample of Fran's placental tissue to a pathology laboratory. It was a long shot. Pathologists aren't sorcerers; they need enough tissue in reasonably good condition. By the time we got Fran's to the lab, little was suitable for meaningful analysis. But we were in luck. Despite the poor quality, we learned that Fran had a rare immune system disorder over and above her known issues. It could be treated if it was detected before it went too far.

In 2008, when this happened, testing for auto-immune problems early in a high-risk pregnancy wasn't as common as it is today, and Fran's issues were of a kind that become conspicuous only during pregnancy, and even then are diagnosable only via appropriate blood tests. So when I read the lab report, I smiled a smile that's unique to doctors, for who else would see anything good in finding that someone has a disease? Before a disease is diagnosed, patient and doctor alike are like soldiers besieged by snipers in the dark, enemies we can't fight because they're unseen. Only when you know who your enemies are and what they're up to can you defend yourself. Now that we knew the identity of the enemy in Fran's body, we were properly equipped to wage war.

The loss of yet another pregnancy, especially one which had seemed at last to be doing well, had left Fran reeling from a blow from which she needed time to recover, but she was far from defeated. The lab finding redoubled her determination. She returned to the IVF clinic and soon conceived anew. This time, she was monitored even more closely by her obstetrician-gynecologist and auto-immune specialist, while I examined her almost weekly. She received anticoagulants, folic acid, aspirin and other anti- inflammatories, lipid emulsion injections and steroids. In line with common practice, her steroids were tapered off around 12 or 13 weeks and lipids a few weeks later, but her intensive examinations continued; with all her doctors now on the alert, when her placental damage began reappearing, we picked it up immediately and responded with instant resumption of steroid treatment, also ordering Fran to bed, rest being a helpful aid to recovery in such circumstances. The placental damage retreated but left little time to rejoice for just as it seemed the war was being won, other battle fronts opened up. At around four months, Fran began bleeding. This was especially terrifying for her as she'd lost her first baby around four months.

She'd been warned that some spotting was likely but this was a lot of blood. An examination revealed it was from a huge clot under the placenta which had become dislodged. Fran was treated for preterm labor with anti-inflammatories and the blood pressure medicine nifedipine, but the rest of the pregnancy was tough. Around 35 weeks, there were signs of umbilical cord compression, random but potentially life-threatening, and it was decided to induce delivery. Her daughter Barbra weighed over four pounds and, despite her early arrival, was both beautiful and healthy. But Fran's story was far from done.

Fast-forward a couple of years. Encouraged by Barbra's robust growth, Fran and Bernard tried to conceive again via IVF. This time it failed, but knowing now that failure is often a temporary setback and a learning experience rather than a sign of an enduring obstacle, they tried again. Fran wasn't on any medication now and hadn't been paying attention to ovulation and menstruation dates, but it had been some time since her last period. While on vacation, without her calendar and not knowing when she'd ovulated, she tried to calculate when her period was going to start so she could tell the fertility specialist when she thought she was ready for her frozen egg transfer. Her IVF doctor and I happened to be on vacation too, but she decided to try working out a few dates to prepare for the IVF. Checking her status on a home pregnancy test kit, she stared at the wand in disbelief. She'd never had a positive test before until she was four weeks pregnant. Now, tantalizingly, the faintest of faint blue shadows appeared on the wand. Could this be? How accurate were these things, anyway? Taking the result at face value, she calculated she was three weeks and four days pregnant. Exhilaration! There was justice in the world!

She came back down to earth fast. Nothing is as sobering as bad memories. A black cloud of negative reasoning engulfed her: given her history, surely she'd lose this one too. She showed Bernard the wand. Forced to choose between optimism and the mistake of getting their hopes up at the cost of another crushing disappointment, he gently suggested that the ghostly blue line might be just a shadow. Best to disregard it and throw the wand in the trash.

Fortunately, there was little time to brood. Not only did they need to focus on getting full value out of their limited vacation time, but their lively daughter had a minor illness needing attention. There was enough going on without obsessing over what might or might not be. Still, Fran couldn't forget what she'd seen. Shadow or not, something had been there. She hadn't imagined it. And with her medical history, if, just if, the line was accurate, there wasn't a moment to waste. Any hope of pregnancy success meant beginning her medication at the very start of the pregnancy, preferably even before ovulation. Conflicted and uncertain, she phoned my office only to hear I was out of the country. She asked for her information to be relayed to me then busied herself with chores while she waited to hear from me. In a while the phone rang with my call from Europe. I prescribed the medication she was to begin taking at once. To her relief, I confirmed she'd acted wisely in tracking me down. It meant the odds were in our favor. Just a short delay would have made us miss the treatment window. A few days later the couple took their still ill toddler to a nearby emergency room; she had flu. Since Bernard remained unconvinced that she was pregnant, Fran asked the ER doctor to give her a blood test. The result was disturbing.

It showed that although technically Fran was pregnant, she had a problematically low level of HCG, human chorionic gonadotropin, a substance known as "the pregnancy hormone". The placenta starts producing it about a week after fertilization. The ER doctor told them that despite the positive pregnancy reading, Fran's HCG level was too low for the pregnancy to be viable. In other words, it was pretty much doomed.

Astoundingly, Fran was undaunted, because although her HCG reading of 250 was below the healthy norm, she understood that the ER doctor was probably measuring her number not against her own history, of which he knew nothing, but against the many other women he routinely examined, who were probably much further along in their pregnancies and therefore would, of course, have much higher HCG numbers. By her standards and history, she reasoned, her number was excellent. She'd seen her earlier number on her home pregnancy kit, indicating that her HCG had doubled in 72 hours, an encouraging sign. It wasn't out blind hope and faith, then, but on the basis of painstakingly gained medical insight that she believed this pregnancy was indeed viable. She left the ER room with optimism that Barbra might well not be an only child.

Fran understood that the coming weeks and months wouldn't be easy. With her pregnancy history, it would be foolish to expect that. She was right. The old enemy thrombophilia again raised its head, and there was clotting. Her immune system problems reasserted themselves and once more necessitated a blend of exactly timed medication and intensive monitoring. There was premature labor and all the suspense and tension that attends the birth of a baby who comes into the world so besieged. But the result was a healthy girl, Irene.

Fran's case ranks as one of my most exasperating and most satisfying. Much of her anguished medical history was explained by the lab analysis of a placental tissue sample so poor in quality it was doubtful the lab would be able to make anything of it. Yet the lab finding made all the difference to Fran's subsequent pregnancy management. This case shows the importance of attention to detail, of preparedness for surprises, and, again, of always examining the placenta promptly after delivery. It's also a tribute to the perinatal pathologists whose skill retrospectively illuminates placental problems despite a prevailing philosophy in today's medical establishment, which minimizes the placenta's role so that thorough pathological investigation of placentas tends to be very rare. Fran's case also highlights, again, how vital timing can be, as well as a mother's persistence, not only against emotional devastation but also in the form of a willingness to endure the unpleasant things that medicines themselves can inflict. Fran's steroid treatments for her immune issues enlarged her neck and cheeks; pimples appeared; hair grew on her neck and face; water pockets ballooned under her armpits. On the plus side, while on steroids, she was rarely tired or nauseated and her enjoyment of all foods increased. (Except for a little weight gain that stayed, her symptoms disappeared after she gave birth.)

In my cases of pregnancy triumph over problems similar to Fran's, all patients had a history of pregnancy loss, all were tested thoroughly before they became pregnant again, and most had clotting disorders affecting placental health. If you're concerned about your ability to sustain a successful pregnancy, get yourself tested for clotting disorders from the outset, preferably before you conceive. My success-story patients have all been monitored every two weeks from the earliest stage with ultrasound and Doppler, treated with low-dose aspirin and, where necessary, injected with the anti-clotting medication LMWH (low-molecular-weight heparin) once or twice daily.

Since I've explained that low PAPP-A indicates clotting problems, it may surprise you that after anti-clotting treatments such patients still had low PAPP-A. To understand why, imagine that a social worker comes across a child whose parents aren't only extremely poor financially but also poorly educated. The social worker sees this as a warning sign that this child, having known only poverty and poor education, needs special encouragement to get a good education, and help to see the connection between poverty and poor education, and that education is a way out of poverty. Now imagine that, with the social worker's support, the child studies hard, wins a scholarship to college and gets a good job. However: none of this will necessarily change the parents. Educationally, they will likely stay pretty much as they were. The warning signal that attracted the social worker's attention (i.e., the condition of the child's parental home), will not necessarily be affected by the cure that is affected in the child. Similarly, in the medical disorder I've just described, neither a warning symptom nor all the conditions causing it will necessarily end after we cure the problem to which the warning signal alerted us.

Also, because of the current limits of our knowledge about the exact relationship between low PAPP-A and the placenta, it's possible (even likely) that some patients whose pregnancies turn out well after the treatment described above might have done well even if they hadn't received those treatments. Who knows? The more important question the patients have to ask is: "How much of a chance do I want to take with my pregnancy?" Generally, if an expectant mother has unexplained low PAPP-A and abnormal ultrasound and Doppler evaluations, I advise starting treatment immediately after drawing blood for coagulation testing, without even waiting for the test result. So commonly do clotting disorders afflict mothers with low PAPP-A, that in the hundreds of my patients who've been treated in this way so far, this confident anticipation of the test result hasn't been wrong even once. Massive evidence confirms compellingly that the sooner we start treatment, the longer and healthier the pregnancy will be. Sufficiently early treatment offers an excellent chance of pregnancy success. Mothers who leave it to 20 weeks before being tested and treated will be lucky if they reach 30 weeks with a healthy baby.

Chapter 19

THE SHOCKING TRUTH ABOUT CARDIOVASCULAR DISEASE IN WOMEN

I have seen in my consulting rooms the consuming anguish of exhausted women whose medical problems impeded their ability to have a baby and who then, perhaps after suffering the traumas of multiple miscarriages, had to face the further strain of hearing from doctors that, oh well, this was just the way things were. And the next step for such a mother is all too often that she concludes her continuing miscarriages, or whatever other painful outcomes the pregnancy complications are causing, are somehow her fault, and that she's simply a failure as a woman. This self-damaging sense of failure is an enormous human problem. The failure is not the mother's but our society's, and particularly the medical establishment's.

As I've said, my patients tend to be not women who struggle to conceive but ones who conceive fairly readily, then face difficulties, sometimes apparently insuperable, in seeing a pregnancy through a full term to a successful birth. Such problems are physiological but their larger context is social. The medical establishment, including the health insurance system, is failing women with poor information about their pregnancy problems and the steps available to fix them. Emotionally, an inability to have a child, when, at a deep level, a woman feels that she can, should and must have one, can be life-altering for both would-be parents. Economically, failing to inform women adequately about how to see a pregnancy through to a successful birth can impose enormous debts on couples who spend money on unnecessarily repeated childbearing efforts. Furthermore, poor information and inappropriate treatments can result in babies born with impairments causing suffering, plus years of expensive medical care and parental stress. Then there's the fact, so little talked about yet crucial to women's well-being, that the information in question is important not only for pregnancy but also for much else in women's health, as I made clear earlier when explaining the Placental Syndrome.

There is a deep-seated failing in the medical establishment's conduct of its public communication responsibilities. This failing can be seen in the astonishing disparity between the amount of money spent on research, advertising, public education and other actions related to breast cancer prevention and treatment, and the funds made available for similar activity in connection with other, even more lethal diseases. As a doctor specializing in women's disorders, I'm fully aware of the toll cancer takes and I appreciate every dime spent on spreading awareness of the facts about cancer, cancer screenings and all else that women should know to avoid this cruel disease. I certainly don't want to see any money subtracted from cancer initiatives. What concerns me is the misleading impression that by targeting any one disorder the providers of funding have somehow discharged our society's obligation to protect women's health. Women aren't stalked by a single medical monster, and achieving great publicity for the war against any one such enemy should not be allowed to distract us from the disgraceful lack of public communication on so vital a subject as the Placental Syndrome. Women's health issues connected with reproductive disorders are being shockingly neglected, and no amount of money spent on appropriately publicizing any other illness should be allowed to obscure this wholly unacceptable fact.

An appalling fact, so little known that it can be regarded as a secret even though anyone can find out about it if they want to, is that every year more American women die of cardiovascular disease than from cancer, accidents, Alzheimer's and respiratory diseases combined. Cardiovascular disease has been well known for many years as the US's leading killer of women beyond the age of menopause.[31, 110-114] Even more horrifying is that we know enough to stop and reverse this trend. However, compared with the public communication efforts devoted to other issues, very scant publicity has been given to the cardiovascular disease crisis. Funding for education to prevent cardiovascular deaths in women is relatively, and for all practical purposes, non-existent. This is a staggering shortcoming in our society's recognition of the medical needs and priorities of women, and a disgraceful, resounding failure of health care policy.

Cardiovascular disease is largely attributable to a number of factors affecting the health of the vascular (blood vessel) lining. The most common is plaque, a deposit formed by a high level of cholesterol, a fatty substance in the blood which is especially damaging when it accumulates under the inner lining of the blood vessels in the heart and brain. (The plaque that collects on our teeth is something else.) We have much yet to learn about cholesterol; for a long time it was thought to come from the cholesterol in our food, but it now appears this isn't so. We know that plaque narrows blood vessels, but in itself it doesn't cause the blockage which leads to heart attack or stroke. This is caused by an increased clotting tendency in the blood. People with normal clotting systems are less likely to have heart attacks and strokes even if there's plaque build-up in their blood vessels.

This relates directly to the Placental Syndrome. Women with this syndrome and women with cardiovascular disease share an abnormal blood clotting tendency, which can lead to restricted blood flow to organs including the heart and brain.[113] Monitoring the placenta enables us not only to spot problems that could damage the pregnancy but also to create a picture of the mother's future health, since placental clotting tendencies provide clues to her likelihood of developing clotting-related problems (including potentially fatal ones) in later years. Also, such pregnancy examinations, conducted properly and to a sufficient extent, can offer early signs of other potential diseases. Pregnancy stress can expose previously undetected physiological abnormalities, even borderline ones, that may become problems; e.g. gestational diabetes. Usually this disorder vanishes after pregnancy, but 60% of patients go on to develop diabetic tendency in later years. And hypertension during pregnancy increases its post-pregnancy likelihood.

While not all ailments experienced during pregnancy resurface in more serious post-pregnancy forms, pregnancy's illumination of physiological weaknesses offers an invaluable map to a healthier future, enabling medical preparation for illnesses that might be worse if they come as surprises. Plainly, then, the job of an obstetrician or maternal-fetal specialist goes (or should go) far beyond seeing a woman through pregnancy. Medical intelligence gained from the womb can powerfully guide health care for years after the pregnancy, regarding diet and other lifestyle choices, with a view to helping women live the longest and healthiest lives they can. Patients whose genes expose them to future diabetes or hypertension can eliminate these vulnerabilities by adjusting their eating habits, controlling their weight and exercising consistently. But this far-reaching scope for health empowerment in light of "womb wisdom" is egregiously absent from the contemporary media spotlight.

Why? For several reasons. One way to interest the media industry in a subject is via big-budget publicity campaigns. The subjects I've discussed above are backed by no such campaigns. Then, the insurance and pharmaceutical industries greatly influence the dissemination of medical information and the behaviors of doctors, and this influence runs counter to the messages I've described. Further, physicians' conservatism tends not to encourage information that rocks the boat. In addition, there's our society's bias favoring male interests. Overwhelmingly, most medical studies on cardiovascular diseases have been primarily on men. While the origins of this imbalance arguably lie in our society's overall gender bias, it was encouraged as doctors increasingly began perceiving female hormones as promoting cardiovascular health. This perception contributed to the idea that women were somehow immune to cardiovascular disease, and that while it wasn't exclusively a men's disease, men suffered most from it; consequently, it became common for cardiovascular studies to focus on males. Fortunately, research on female cardiovascular disorders continued despite these handicaps, and eventually, it became clear that women's risk of death from cardiovascular disease increased significantly after menopause until it exceeded the risk of men of like age. Many studies indicate that over 30% of women die of cardiovascular disease after menopause, while deaths from breast cancer don't exceed 2% (although the lifelong risk that women will develop some form of breast cancer is about 10%).

Fairly recent efforts have begun to correct the cardiovascular research imbalance, but generations of prejudice isn't quickly reversed. Gender bias is deeply entrenched in our civilization, arguably even influencing some nuances of feminism so that efforts to recognize the unique female identity can be paradoxically expressed as a campaign to make women more like men, a trend which surely can't promote a fuller appreciation of motherhood. One of the most pressing challenges of our time is to achieve an equality of gender rights which accurately reflects gender identities. Future historians may marvel at the misguided finding, in our day, of political satisfaction in pretending that women and men are pretty much the same and that possessing a womb is a superficiality. Often in the delivery room, holding a newborn whose mother had persisted with her pregnancy after miscarriages and other disasters which would cow the strongest men, I've felt in the presence of a strength of determination seemingly beyond flesh and blood, beside which the powers of my male sex looked frail. In such a mother's eyes, half-closed by medication and exhaustion, I've glimpsed flashes of the same distant fire, it seemed to me, that our imaginations call feebly into the mind's eye when we look up at the stars. To objections that I'm overdramatizing an everyday biological event, my response is that if you'd participated in thousands of births as I have, and not just conventional births, which are astonishing enough but deliveries that consummated voyages in which mother and unborn child have for long months together suspensefully navigated one looming catastrophe after another, you too would emerge from the theaters of such desperate battles for life feeling that you've looked into the heart of a strength greater than human minds can hold. What a strange irony that our proud civilization, aspiring to grand adventures in space, seems so uncomfortable facing forces greater than the men who've traditionally ruled it, and beyond their personal male experience, so that there is a common impulse to tiptoe around both the awesome imperatives of motherhood and the burdens and vulnerabilities to which they expose women. It's as if, in its unease with the powers that reside within womanhood, our gender-biased society wants women to pay for their identity through the exaction from them of punitive taxes, in ways which include a withholding of funding for public education about female medical needs. These circumstances are vital to women who experience high-risk pregnancy. Because studies indicate that women who experience pregnancy complications are significantly likelier to die from cardiovascular disease than from all other causes combined, my daily work with women struggling through high-risk pregnancies have convinced me that it is essential for all women to be made urgently aware of the perils of cardiovascular disease on the two fronts that I've described: the threat that such disease poses to all post-menopausal women, and its danger to women who are trying to sustain a pregnancy in the face of medical complications. These two linked areas of hazard form a continuous landscape of neglect, and we should all feel and express outrage that our society disgracefully glosses over the high death rate among women from cardiovascular disease both in later life and during high-risk pregnancies. So little information is publicly circulated about these shocking conditions that it's hard to find women, even in highly educated circles, who have heard of cardiovascular disease as a subject of importance to their gender. It's as if this information, which is of such life-and-death significance to women across the age spectrum, is regarded as being not worth the time of medical health publicists, advertisers, media practitioners, public health policymakers, public education funders, and leaders of the medical establishment. Like the Placental Syndrome, this issue is one of our society's blind spots.

Now, we've seen that too much clotting blocks and damages blood vessels, and, as the placenta is a vascular organ, this is bad news for a fetus. On the other hand, too little clotting is also dangerous: abnormally thin blood causes excessive bleeding, which might issue spontaneously from your nose, stomach, kidneys or any other organ, or even a slight wound can bleed without stopping. You've probably heard of hemophilia, a group of genetic disorders interfering with the body's ability to regulate blood clotting. Unless they're treated with corrective medicine, people with this condition are at high risk of bleeding to death if they get hurt, or even during surgery. I've discussed, on the other hand, people whose blood clots too much or too easily have thrombophilia. What I haven't yet explained is that thrombophilia arises when your blood has too much of a substance called factor VIII. (This is always spelled with Roman numerals rather than as factor 8.) At the same time, your blood contains natural blood-thinning chemicals, including one called protein S, and, if your blood has too little of this, then you'll also be at increased risk of clotting. There are more chemicals involved in clotting, but I'm not going to go into them all; I've mentioned the ones above only to emphasize that clotting problems usually happen because of a chemical imbalance: too little of one chemical or too much of another. A serious imbalance tends to be caused by either one big problem of this kind or by multiple small problems popping up more or less simultaneously. When multiple problems are at work, it's harder to diagnose them by blood tests because the test may focus on a single chemical which may not be at such an abnormal level that it causes an alarming result. It's only when it's seen in the broader context of other problems that its importance becomes apparent. As I noted earlier, a major challenge in understanding pregnancy problems is that so much is connected. The broader context of a problem can be invisible unless a doctor looks specifically for it. For example: blood levels of protein S and another key chemical, protein C, can be low but still in the normal range and yet, nevertheless, signify serious risk of excessive clotting in the placenta if they're combined with also normal but low levels of a substance called antithrombin III. Mothers with such "normal" borderline test readings sometimes don't receive proper treatment because they're seen as technically in normal range, even though the appearance of the separate readings together indicate a potentially serious abnormality. Many such mothers have gone on to experience pregnancy disasters after their doctors evaluated them for thrombophilia and pronounced that all was well. Then, when the pregnancy turned bad, it was called an "unexplained" outcome. To make matters worse, such patients will often still not be treated properly when they become pregnant again.

 The diagnostic limitations of today's pregnancy management are well illustrated by doctors' handling of thrombophilia's genetic background. Many doctors tend to disregard some genetic information that can signal potentially serious problems. A major problem is that instead of studying the mother's overall medical profile, they see risk factors in isolation. But, here again, it's how those factors can work together that's crucial. Evidence indicates that two or more minor factors can have graver pregnancy consequences than one major factor.[115] For instance, many doctors looking for thrombophilia risks in pregnancy will focus on whether one of the mother's legs has a clot in a major vein. If such a clot makes its way to a lung (where it's called a pulmonary embolism) and is big enough, it can be deadly. This single-minded preoccupation with a big blood clot in one area of the body is common among blood specialists (hematologists), whose mostly older patients are prone to this kind of problem and related issues, like strokes. The trouble is, many hematologists don't know much about the placenta, pregnancy management or fetal development. These subjects don't form a major part of their training or professional practice. They rarely see pregnant mothers. On the other hand, most perinatologists (obstetricians who specialize in maternal-fetal medicine) aren't currently trained in clotting disorders, so when they encounter a pregnancy complicated by such a disorder, they naturally enough refer the patient to a hematologist. See the circle? The perinatologist, whose forte isn't clotting, sends the patient to a hematologist who lacks placental knowledge. The result tends not to be one expert compensating for the other's lack of expertise but rather two areas of ignorance uniting to create a more dangerous one. This situation shouldn't exist in health care but it does, and it illustrates further why you as a mother, and not the medical establishment, must own your pregnancy assertively and be ultimately responsible for its management. Hematologists have invaluable expertise, gained through arduous training, and

I certainly mean no disrespect toward them when I tell you that placental clotting is too important to be left to a hematologist. It must be handled by an experienced maternal-fetal specialist who understands both clotting and placental circulation.

Clotting issues vary in both likelihood and level of danger. Severely low protein S, antithrombin III or protein C can by themselves cause significant clotting for baby and mother, as can the genetic conditions called factor V Leiden and factor II. Factor V, the commonest of the rare genetic conditions, affects up to (depending on which population segment we're talking about) 15% percent of people with Mediterranean ancestry and 3% to 5% of African Americans. Factor II and other severe conditions occur in 1% to 2% of all pregnancies. Protein S deficiency affects about 25% of all mothers yet is commonly undiagnosed or ignored. Unless it's diagnosed before pregnancy, the standard of care is to dismiss it as an unproblematic feature of pregnancy requiring no action. This is a momentous mistake. While most initially low protein S levels do re-enter normal range after pregnancy and may not then pose a risk to the mother, during pregnancy, they can damage the placenta, thus harming the baby.

The story of gestational diabetes has been similar. Several decades ago, it was discovered that blood sugar could rise during pregnancy, causing a temporary diabetes which disappeared as the sugar level returned to normal after birth. This was initially seen as a normal pregnancy condition requiring no action. Only after many fetal deaths did doctors realize they should aggressively treat gestational diabetes and gestational hypertension. Just because an abnormality goes away after pregnancy doesn't make it safe during pregnancy. The same holds true for all gestational clotting disorders. The lesson is, again, that the placenta must be monitored, because only reassurance that it's on a healthy development path will allow a well-peace of mind regarding any pregnancy at risk of clotting problems. If there's any evidence at all of placental clotting damage the mother MUST be treated to protect the baby.

Gestational immune-system clotting problems usually involve those malfunctioning antibodies that have featured in earlier pages. These objects interfere with phospholipids, fat-derived substances that make up much of the membranes of your body's cells. Phospholipids normally help regulate clotting. When rogue antibodies get in the way of this job, there are disastrous results for the placenta. Think about it: the lining of the placenta's intervillous space, that meeting area where your blood gives your baby food and oxygen and removes waste, is a cell membrane. So if rogue antibodies prevent the phospholipids from servicing cell membranes properly, your placenta is in the direct line of fire. Yet the current standard of care is to test for such problems only after pregnancy because the prevailing custom is that gestational thrombophilia should be ignored!

The wide applicability of some of the facts I'm explaining must never be allowed to obscure the overriding uniqueness of every placenta and its ways of responding to challenges. The importance of placental individuality has been confirmed repeatedly by my clinical experiences. For example, I've known several cases of twin pregnancies with antibody problems where one placenta was badly damaged and the other wasn't. To me, this strongly suggests that a mother's immune system interacts differently with each fetus. This makes sense, since each baby is genetically unique. It also explains why not all pregnancies with these problems will necessarily end badly. Mild immune-system clotting abnormality may cause minimal placental damage. But the damage can also be so severe that the baby will die. Twin pregnancies show dramatically how placentas that provoke the mother's immune system are more likely to be attacked by it. This capacity to provoke, shaped by genetics, is one of the reasons why it always makes sense to look for signals from the placenta to help decide if treatment is necessary. Where clotting problems arise from gestational immune problems, the outcomes are better when they're treated consistently. Mothers who aren't treated consistently have random outcomes, sometimes successful and sometimes not. Proper monitoring and consistent treatment can reduce and even eliminate the randomness. A study that compared placentas whose antibody problems had been detected before pregnancy with placentas whose problems were detected during pregnancy (with a normal antibody test result after birth) found that all the placentas had the same degree and kind of clotting. Thus, distinguishing between the two timeframes of antibody problem detection, for management and treatment purposes, is meaningless. This finding probably won't bring about a new standard of care because of the medical establishment's position that changes in the standard of care can be justified only on the basis of expensive further studies which, in this case, seem highly unlikely to be funded. I believe such studies aren't needed, given the abundant clinical-practice-based evidence that "gestational only" anti-phospholipid antibodies are in fact dangerous to pregnancy. But currently, this evidence will be used to save lives only if it's applied by doctors who are willing to buck the prevailing trend, and if enough readers talk, via social media and other means, about the information I'm setting out in this book.

Chapter 20

THE FATHER'S STORY

One of the oddest (and most potent) failures in the medical establishment's handling of placental clotting is insufficient appreciation of the fact that a baby has two parents.

Of course everyone knows that a baby has a mother and a father. But by "appreciation" of this fact, I'm talking about understanding the genetic implications of this dual parenthood. Most clotting conditions can be traced back to a faulty parental gene. For some reason, however, most perinatologists associate genetic thrombophilia with only the mother. This error contributes to the deaths of thousands of otherwise healthy fetuses.

In genetic thrombophilia, the father as well as the mother can pass thrombophilia on to the baby, and if the father has thrombophilia he may well be unaware of it. In half of all fetal deaths from genetic thrombophilia, the father is the main problem. I say "main" because the baby's inheritance from the father can be worsened by the mother's genes, which can cause her to have non-genetic but still problematic thrombophilia, immune thrombophilia, which won't be transmitted to the baby but will still affect it because it can most definitely damage the placenta. The baby is affected by thrombophilia whether the cause is genetic or non-genetic. Yet, as if it weren't strange enough that fathers are commonly left out of the thrombophilia equation, stranger still is the fact that babies are also left out of it.[116-120]

Treating any thrombophilia as something that affects only the mother is an approach that has no basis in physiological reality. Nevertheless, this approach is frighteningly widespread. Because studies of thrombophilia are still relatively new to the textbooks used in medical training, many doctors don't know a fetus can have thrombophilia. So usually, only the mother is tested for it. This contributes significantly to the high incidence of recurrent miscarriage. But I want to stress that even genetic thrombophilia can't entirely destroy your chances of a good pregnancy. In principle, because each pregnancy is unique, a mother who tries long enough has at least some chance of achieving a good pregnancy even with problematic genes from both parents. Every person's genetic inheritance is like a deck of playing cards. The more you try, the better your chances of being dealt a good hand. This is, after all, how we all got here over thousands of years of evolution despite the limited medical knowledge available over most of our history as a species. But there's more to it even than the hand you're dealt. As any good card-player will tell you, the outcome of your game depends not only on your hand but on how you play it, and playing well today means using every bit of clinical knowledge you can lay your hands on, taking into account all the factors that can raise your risk profile, including your age.

As we've seen, age matters, and given that many causes of recurrent miscarriage are age-related, it's unsurprising that the risk of genetic defects, too, increases with a mother's age, as does the severity of thrombophilia, which causes almost two-thirds of recurrent miscarriages. The fact that women used to start having babies as soon as they could and didn't stop until menopause meant that, although many babies were lost, enough made it to keep us going as a species. If every couple manages to have three healthy babies, the population doubles every two generations. But today we face not only a drastically smaller pregnancy opportunity window (with most women not voluntarily attempting pregnancy until their 30s after completing education and establishing a career foothold) but also, to make things worse, the fact that advancing maternal age is associated with declining fertility. The change in child-bearing age is therefore not just a sociological revolution but also a biological one whose implications are far from universally recognized by either the medical community or the public. Until this changes, women will continue unnecessarily to suffer complicated pregnancies including ones that end in either one-time or recurrent miscarriage. And here again I mention the shortcomings of the medical profession because while my primary aim in this book is to inform you, I'm also hoping that by informing you, I'll be able, with your help, to help others beyond this book's readers. This can be achieved if you talk to your doctor and also to your friends, via social media or in any other way, about what I'm sharing with you here; spreading the word will help, I believe, to influence the medical establishment to cure some of the problems that exist within the establishment itself regarding pregnancy management and especially placental care.

In my work dealing with pregnancy complications, I've often wished that, before they came to me and were being seen by other physicians, patients had been given the information I've been setting out. Not only would this have helped me to explain to them what ailed them and the thinking behind my treatments, but that knowledge may even have made it unnecessary for them to come to me at all. This applies particularly strongly to thrombophilia. It's my impression that while more and more doctors have been coming to recognize, on the basis of clinical experience, that thrombophilia causes a significant number of pregnancy complications and bad outcomes, many more doctors refuse to accept this, due to long-established habit and the herd mentality.

In view of all this you might wonder: if medicine is so opinion-driven, is it really scientific? This is a good question which I'll answer as best as I can. From one perspective, the institutional collection of medical observations, the construction of theories to explain that data, and the measuring of those theories against clinical experience certainly amounts to a scientific endeavor. In this sense, medicine brings together disciplines like chemistry, which enables us to make predictions of how substances behave in various circumstances, and anatomy, which describes the parts of the body and how they work together. Such disciplines, which contribute to the foundation of clinical practice, are undeniably sciences, and give medicine a firmly scientific basis. We've amassed an enormous number of hard facts about the biological, chemical, physical and even mathematical foundations of medicine that enable us to make exact measurements of phenomena, control events in laboratories and make highly accurate predictions in many instances. This fund of medical knowledge is definitely scientific in its exactness and the rigor of the methods by which it's obtained, verified, systematized and periodically updated.

The practice of medicine, on the other hand, is a different matter. This involves using scientific information in a clinical situation, where the doctor works not only with facts drawn from the scientific disciplines I've mentioned, but also with information gathered from clinical interactions with patients, drawing on judgment, experience and philosophical approach and the patient's test results, symptoms, communications and behavior. Every human individual is vastly complex and the interactions between two human individuals (such as patient and doctor) takes this complexity to an even greater level, which is then magnified further by the relationships that each of those two individuals has with other individuals, and by the histories of those relationships and the influences that have been brought to bear on them from many sources, such as logical reasoning, personal experience, education and training, culture, social and economic background, religious and philosophical beliefs, political inclinations, personality, and more. In this larger setting I can't see how medical practice can plausibly be called a science, because although laboratories support the things that physicians do, patients themselves are not laboratory specimens and their problems don't unfold in the artificial environments of laboratories but in the messy reality of life, which is shot through with subjective and unknown factors requiring guesswork, intuition and the wisdom that comes from hands-on experience. Much medical practice involves a multi-nuanced dialogue between doctor and patient in the context of the emotional and philosophical bonds that each one has with many other people and institutions outside the doctor's consulting room, including the doctor's professional relationships with medical power structures (such as insurance companies) which influence how a doctor selects, interprets and applies knowledge in any given case.

 The facts of thrombophilia form part of this landscape of intangible human forces, as do other controversies related to pregnancy. With regard to pregnancy-related clotting problems, for example, relatively few doctors are familiar with the gene mutations MTHFR, 4G/5G (also known as PAI-1) and ACE insertion/deletion mutations. The MTHFR mutation affects the fetus and the placenta in several ways, while the 4G/5G gene, which many obstetricians have never heard of, regulates the body's ability to break down clots; a fault in it can cause complete failure of embryo implantation. In milder forms it can impair the takeover and conversion of spiral arteries, which as we've seen is crucial to the health of the placenta and to the baby's supply of food and oxygen. This genetic malfunction can also cause placenta accreta, a condition resulting in excessive bleeding after delivery because the placenta can't be removed from the uterus in the normal way. (Hysterectomy is common in these cases.) The same gene fault can cause insulin problems leading to diabetes as well as ovarian cysts, inability to ovulate properly, and hypofibrinolysis, a weakened ability to break down clots.[121] Because of a widespread lack of training and information about this spectrum of disorders ("4G/5G gene polymorphism-derived problems") it's common for obstetricians to treat patients only during the first trimester. This means the treatment is geared to preventing abortion but not to achieving a healthy pregnancy. Hypofibrinolysis can harm the placenta throughout the entire length of a full-term pregnancy.

The ACE insertion/deletion gene mutation, one of the most neglected gene disorders, can catastrophically impair the spiral artery remodeling and cause thickening of the walls of fetal-placental blood vessels, leading to preterm births, severe fetal growth retardation, pre-eclampsia and recurrent pregnancy loss, all of which arise from defective placenta development.[122] ACE-mutation mothers' risk of hypertension is significantly higher.

THE FATHER'S STORY

Considerable clinical experience shows that ACE should be treated like any other clotting condition in pregnancy, i.e. with aspirin and LMWH (low-molecular-weight heparin) in the right doses at the right moment in the pregnancy, plus close ultrasound and Doppler monitoring for proper placental development, as well as cervical evaluation to detect premature cervical shortening and prevent preterm delivery. This approach, along with testing for ACE and other gene disorders sufficiently early, can significantly reduce the risk of pregnancy loss and other bad outcomes. Yet it's unusual for these things to be done.[123, 124]

We've seen, then, that many genetic factors cause clotting or are associated with it; these include low levels of protein S, protein C and antithrombin III (these all being associated with preterm birth, placental thrombosis, pre-eclampsia and other placental complications), as well as high levels of factors VIII (associated with increased risk for thrombosis, recurrent pregnancy loss and other placental complications), XI, IX, XII and XIII (these latter are also associated with recurrent pregnancy loss). But as important as these genetic problems are, the diversity of non-genetic problems deserves no less attention. The rogue antibodies, e.g., come in different varieties and can be triggered in varied ways. Annexin V, a substance located in the inner lining of the placenta, protects the placenta from excessive clotting, but anti-annexin V antibodies can inhibit this function, causing clotting in the intervillous space by helping the clotting substance fibrin to accumulate on the surface of the chorionic villi, thickening the membrane barrier between the maternal and fetal blood, making it harder for food and oxygen to reach the fetus, which can lead to recurrent pregnancy loss, infertility and the failure of in vitro fertilization treatment.

The womb is a busy, busy place.

Other antibodies can interfere with the normal function of platelets, those small structures in the blood which are involved in clotting. This can hamper embryo and placenta development and contribute to recurrent pregnancy loss. About 22% of all recurrent pregnancy loss is associated with "sticky platelet syndrome," which causes excessive placental clotting. Aspirin, in the right doses at the right times, is the best treatment. Then there's plasmin, a natural anti-clotting substance in your blood. Sometimes a chemical called alpha2-antiplasmin develops, interfering with plasmin and so increasing the risk of abnormal clotting. Then, the clotting substance fibrinogen is commonly increased during pregnancy but, if the level gets too high, abnormal clotting can result, while the fatty chemical lipoprotein (a) can cause bad clotting-related problems and is associated with increased risk of bad pregnancy outcomes, and protein Z deficiency is associated with a raised risk of severe placental problems happening soon after the mother's and fetus's blood circulations become linked; it's associated with pre-eclampsia, fetal growth problems, fetal death and recurrent unexplained pregnancy loss. Protein Z deficiency in combination with the factor V gene mutation is associated with severe clotting issues: together these conditions can be lethal.[125-127]

It's very hard to judge exactly how to treat and manage a pregnancy with clotting complications. There's good scope to be either insufficiently sensitive to the many risks or to be overprotective. A good guiding principle is to be overprotective of your pregnancy rather than run the risk of being underprotective, given the possibly lethal consequences of many clotting problems. These potential consequences, by the way, include clotting in the mother after the pregnancy: the two weeks after birth are the most dangerous for this as the mother's clotting system is then superactive, creating a serious risk of DVT (deep vein thrombosis), especially in the legs. Substantial evidence indicates that all mothers with clotting problems, even minor ones, should be treated with LMWH in these critical two weeks. A patient of mine who declined this treatment developed both DVT and pulmonary embolism (a clot in the lung) and she had to go on long-term anti-clotting medication to avoid life-threatening repercussions.

The most complex single factor in all these clotting problems is the profoundly close physiological relationship between mother and baby. Much of the medical profession's murky understanding of clotting is tied up with an insufficient appreciation of this relationship's complexity. For instance, consider the mistaken idea that placental thrombosis originates only or principally in the mother's circulation. This belief continues to be common among doctors despite massive evidence to the contrary dating back to the 1930s, with confirmations dating from the 1980s and after.[35, 37, 119, 128-131] This is one of the tragedies of contemporary medicine. Of course, the mother's circulation is not irrelevant. Maternal diabetes, hypertension, immune system disorders and other problems can certainly be an initial cause of placental thrombosis. But compelling evidence shows that the vast majority of placental thrombosis cases originate in the circulation of fetuses whose mothers' circulations are quite healthy. In case after case, such pregnancies' clotting problems have clearly been due to placental disorders. It's even been documented that the mother's circulation can remain fine up to two weeks after the complete degeneration of the placental villi. If all this seems complicated, that's because it is! Although becoming pregnant is a complex process shaped by many things, even greater complexity seems to attend the enormous number of factors that determine whether the pregnancy will be healthy and full-term. This is why we must engage with the full spectrum of factors that can impact the placenta, instead of being content (as many doctors are) just to test the mother's blood. While nobody wants to see tests conducted without good reason, the current trend is in the opposite direction: too many doctors conduct insufficient tests. This explains why so many pregnancy losses and bad outcomes are conveniently written off as "unexplained." Proper placental monitoring with appropriate testing enables us not only to explain many problems but also, frequently, to prevent them from becoming large enough to damage the baby. At the very least, the right testing at the right time often yields enough information to protect the next pregnancy. Yet extensive clinical records show that many patients lose more than five pregnancies before they are properly tested.

Here are two key insights which have been repeatedly validated by the successful treatment of thousands of patients and all known varieties of clotting defects: (1) Never underestimate the complexity of clotting, its causes and its impact on the placenta; and (2) Always listen to the placenta. Monitor it, shape your pregnancy management around what your placenta tells you about its health at every stage, and you'll be on solid ground.

Chapter 21

FEAR OF LAWSUITS, AND THE POLITICS OF MOTHERHOOD

Clinical evidence shows that, by treating the placenta, it's possible either to restore lost portions of placental tissue or at least prevent the spread of placental damage. When any placental thrombosis or fetal thrombotic damage is noticed, the first priority is to use Doppler scanning to learn whether the mother's circulation serving the damaged area is OK. If the maternal circulation is intact and continues to supply the empty intervillous space, adjusting the anticoagulant treatment (either increasing the dose or increasing the frequency of injections to twice daily) can in many cases restore the damaged tissue by stimulating new chorionic villi growth. Heparin and LMWH aren't only anticoagulants; all heparin-based anticoagulants suppress NK cell activity as well as the excessive molecules called cytokines that, in many cases, cause inflammation and thrombotic problems in fetal blood vessels.[132, 133] (Sometimes the immune system turns some white blood cells into macrophages, objects which digest sick and dead matter. Cytokines are created as a by-product of this digestion process. Too many of them can cause various types of damage including to the cervix, as we'll see later.) Furthermore, heparins are angiogenic, i.e. they stimulate growth of new blood vessels in the chorionic villi.[134] Angiogenesis is the first step in enlarging and expanding the villous network.

Despite the significant knowledge that it can reduce or stop placental damage, enabling the womb to regain stable activity, this placenta-focused treatment approach remains widely unfashionable among doctors, largely because of its relative unfamiliarity. The price for this mistake is meanwhile being paid by mothers and babies. The questionableness of important aspects of prevailing obstetric practice is illustrated further by the examples of magnesium sulfate and terbutaline. Many obstetricians have in the past used these two drugs, and some still do, to try to stop premature labor, despite their having been shown to be ineffective as well as dangerous to both mother and baby. Strangely, doctors who use these obsolete drugs may be among the same doctors who will tell you there's no evidence supporting the use of LMWH to treat patients with placental thrombosis. Similarly, many doctors reject cervical cerclage (stitching) because of alleged lack of evidence about its safety, despite its having been used safely for over half a century! You can see from these instances how obstinately doctors can dig their heels in to avoid the discomfort of having to change their accustomed ways regardless of evidence. There's certainly no shortage of evidence to validate everything I've been telling you about clotting, e.g. that bleeding any time in a pregnancy is bad, that 75% of pregnancies with any abnormal clotting anywhere in the uterus result in miscarriage,[135-138] fetal death, preterm birth, placenta abruptio, pre-eclampsia, growth restriction, cerebral palsy or other fetal brain damage, and/or the baby's death after birth.[139, 140] Moreover, substantial evidence makes it clear that no safety issues arise in any of the treatments I've described, none of which involve drugs known to have potentially damaging side effects like those associated with cancer chemotherapy. Aspirin and heparin have long, well-documented histories. The only concern anyone could possibly have about them is that a patient who's injured while taking them might bleed excessively. Accidents likely to cause excessive bleeding are rare, though. To put this level of risk into statistical perspective, consider this. In theory, a mother could die as a result of having a cesarean section, but this happens only once in about 5000 cesareans, which means the same mother would have double the risk of getting killed just by crossing the street in New York City, where I live. Like millions of others, I cross the street without concern, confident that reasonable precautions will protect me, and the same applies to taking blood-thinners, and, for that matter, all medicine: just ensure that you take the right dose at the right time, with appropriate medical advice. I have yet to meet any patient whose pregnancy treatment experience contradicts this statement.

Knowing how anti-clotting medication works helps one see how baseless the fears are. Aspirin works like a police officer going around your bloodstream preventing blood platelets from sticking to each other (such sticking activates clotting). Aspirin's effect on any platelet lasts for the platelet's entire lifespan of around 10 days. If you take the right dose of aspirin today, all your platelets will be affected. But, every day, about a 10th of your platelets die and are replaced by new platelets, which will be unaffected by aspirin. The right intake of aspirin will thus give your blood an effective balance between protection against excessive clotting and protection against excessive bleeding. The anti-clotting medication heparin (the ordinary kind, not low-molecular-weight heparin) affects platelets differently, and a recommended dose lasts just two to four hours. In rare cases, a patient can have a reaction against heparin. Most effects of this kind are mild and can be stopped swiftly just by discontinuing heparin. In even rarer cases, the reaction may be extreme enough to pose a potential danger, by reducing the number of active platelets so much as to cause excessive bleeding; this is a difficult problem requiring additional anticoagulation treatment with potentially risky new drugs. Low-molecular-weight heparin (LMWH), on the other hand, is even safer than aspirin and ordinary heparin because it counteracts clotting without affecting the platelets. Despite this, many doctors refuse to use it, or don't use it appropriately, for fear that it may cause abnormal bleeding around the spine in patients who receive epidural anesthesia (a local injection of pain-dulling drugs around the lower spine during labor), or spinal anesthesia for any surgery. This has happened to some patients, yes. But a culture of grossly disproportionate anxiety has been created around this medication by drug companies who like to shift lawsuit liability from themselves to doctors. This is common in the pharmaceutical industry, especially for pregnancy medications. Here are some facts.

The LMWH scaremongers have cited a study that showed increased risk for patients undergoing spinal anesthesia in women aged 66 and up.[141] How many pregnant women do you know in that age group? And some people of that age can bleed if they're just touched, regardless of what medicine they've taken. Elderly folk often have black and blue marks. These are caused by age-related weakness of the clotting system along with fragile tissues. The same vulnerability doesn't apply to women in their 30s having a baby. Nevertheless, by surrounding LMWH with legal warnings to satisfy their lawyers and money managers, the drug companies have paralyzed many doctors with a fear of being sued if they use this valuable medication, however carefully, appropriately and beneficially. Because of this fear, many anesthesiologists refuse to give epidural anesthesia to a woman in labor if she's been on LMWH in the preceding 48 hours. This absurd alarmism is a huge disservice to women and is allowing America's lawsuit culture and financial interests to prevent physicians from fulfilling their responsibilities to their patients. It's a well-documented fact that no trace of LMWH remains in a mother's blood 12 hours after the last injection of it.[142, 143] There's no medical reason to deny epidural anesthesia to such a patient. Moreover, epidural anesthesia (when part of a conscious patient's body is numbed) is much safer than general anesthesia (when the patient is unconscious). So there are good medical grounds to use epidural anesthesia even less than 12 hours after the last LMWH shot. The patient can usually be injected with protamine sulfate, which neutralizes at least two-thirds of the LMWH effects. The only mothers who should receive general anesthesia are ones who just received LMWH and have to be anesthetized immediately, and, furthermore, who happen to have some condition that makes protamine sulfate unsuitable for them. Such a patient would be rare indeed. The right thing to do, medically and morally, is to make LMWH and epidural anesthesia available to all mothers who need them. But the opposite is being done. A combination of ignorance and fear of being sued has resulted in many patients being forced into general anesthesia with all its real risks. The word "ignorance" here isn't meant to insult anyone in the medical profession, to which I belong and from which the clinical information in this book comes. I use the word "ignorance" in its straightforward factual sense, meaning a lack of knowledge. For example, it's solidly established that for all practical purposes the effects of ordinary heparin are gone four hours after injection, so when anesthesiologists tell patients not to take heparin 48 hours before surgery, their advice is based on a lack of knowledge. When an anxious patient reports to me her anesthesiologist's unwillingness to provide professional service if she took heparin in the past two days, it's clear to me that the anesthesiologist needs counseling and help to understand that both ordinary heparin and LMWH are quite safe when administered by a well-informed doctor, with LMWH being superior to heparin. If anyone tells you otherwise, ask to see what evidence they have. Base your pregnancy care on science, not superstition.

There is a figure of speech whereby, if you want to describe a battle in its most powerfully waged form, you say that the battle has now "become personal." That is, the fight has reached a stage where it's touched the fighter's innermost personal values, dignity, sense of rightness, and resolve. Physiologically, of course, the pregnancy experience is and has always been intensely personal for women, whom it subjects to far-reaching physical changes and challenges of body and spirit. That is true even of the most straightforward pregnancies and much more fiercely in complicated pregnancies, with their enormously magnified stresses. But I see little appreciation of the great cultural battle that pregnant women also have to be prepared to wage on a personal level. It's in part precisely because the physical struggle is taken so much for granted that the cultural struggle is overlooked. Modern women are in large measure prisoners of a prevailing culture of pregnancy, which cruelly extends the other constraints imposed on women in the past and the present.

There is in our society a deep-rooted idea that to undergo physical trials during pregnancy is a woman's lot. Pregnancy, so it's stated or intimated, along with everything and anything that it may exact from a woman, is simply a fact of life beyond questioning. However: while it's true that biology has assigned motherhood to women, nowhere in our biological architecture is it written that motherhood requires a woman to do whatever society demands of her. Yet throughout history, cultures around the world have imposed penalties on women because of their procreative function. Women have been treated unfairly for generations, in workplaces and elsewhere, simply because they happened to possess bodies which evolution has made essential to our collective survival. We are today the inheritors of that legacy of prejudice against motherhood. When I say expectant mothers contending with complicated pregnancies must be prepared for a fight that will get personal, I'm talking about this cultural battle against prejudice, in which not only the dignity and rights of women but their health and even their lives, as well as the lives of their unborn, depend. There is a culture of deeply ingrained prejudice against mothers who refuse to accept that pregnancy disasters, including one miscarriage after another, are just realities of feminine life which women must uncomplainingly accept. This culture, extending into the very medical profession which is supposed to protect women and their babies, is not ordained by biology. It is a social construct against which the time has come to rebel. This is what I mean when I speak of the fight getting personal, and of women having to take ownership of their bodies and pregnancies back from medical practitioners and medical insurance companies. Why should the customs of these institutions inflict suffering on women and cost the lives of babies for no other reason than that such circumstances suit the convenience, financial and otherwise, of the medical establishment?

As I noted earlier, my own career as a physician specializing in complicated pregnancies has led me to get personal in ways I never dreamed of when I began my medical training. I never suspected that my work as a doctor would lead me one day to become committed, as I am now, to a cultural struggle against the medical establishment's attitudes about pregnancy and the right of women to obtain the care that they and their unborn babies deserve. I'm a member of that community of Americans who are so much in the news these days: immigrants. I was born in Greece at a time when America's place in the world was very different from what it is as I write this. In the decades after World War II, the United States continued to be regarded as the nation which, working with its allies, defeated Nazi Germany, which had ruinously occupied my own homeland. Although the war in Vietnam affected its image at home and abroad, America was admired by millions in many countries as a haven of freedom and standard-bearer of democracy, enlightenment and human rights, and as the country to which the best energies of the world naturally tended to gravitate. In the summer of 1974, when I was a 4th-year medical student, I was selected by one of my professors, along with other five students, to spend three months participating in cutting-edge research of my choice at the University of California, San Francisco. I chose to work with early mouse embryos, flushing them out of their mother's oviduct and raising them in test tubes until their hearts started beating. This exhilarating experience lit a ferocious fire in my heart to make every effort to come back and further my studies in such a scientifically advanced research environment.

To Europeans of my generation, America was a glittering marvel of civilization. To many of us, its materialism and obsession with money, unashamedly broadcast in its movies and other cultural products, was already a cause for wariness, but these reservations were transcended by America's omnipresent vitality, which seemed to rest on an unquenchable national hunger for quality, not only of consumer products but of endeavor and professional expertise and integrity, whether in business, science, art or public service, so that to be an American seemed to be the luckiest status in the world. When I returned to America after completing my initial medical studies in Greece, I stepped on to the soil of my new country full of awe and gratitude at having been granted the gift of good fortune to come and further my studies in so miraculous a place. Here, the best and brightest could be found, and the world's most learned came to pool their knowledge. How inconceivable it would have been to me in those days if some prophet had told me that my progress through the American medical profession, and my years of practice with desperate patients seeking only to see their babies born safely and well, would lead me to become a maverick among maternal-fetal specialists. How bizarre a piece of mischief-making it would have seemed to me if I had heard that one day I would be a critic of my profession, even to the extent of passing up prestigious academic opportunities in leading institutions because I could no longer in good conscience associate myself with the teachings about medicine, and especially pregnancy medicine and management, that were accepted in the highest professional circles despite their being contradicted by my steadily increasing clinical experience.

To my surprise I was to become convinced that these accepted medical customs were wrong, and that the well-being of women and the health and even the lives of their unborn babies were being sacrificed as a result. As the years passed, what I learned from my work with many thousands of patients made me an outsider in my profession. I found myself in disagreement with distinguished and influential peers and, more unnervingly, with mighty corporate interests whose executives didn't take kindly to a maternal-fetal specialist breaking ranks to walk his own path and treat his patients along lines which deviated from the official collective line. The phenomenon of outsiders has always been with us and no doubt always will be, because it is in the nature of new ideas to begin with individuals and small groups who oppose prevailing attitudes; from these small beginnings, new concepts expand outwards, winning over supporters until the mainstream adopts them. This is how ideas evolve in all fields including medicine. It is a process that can be hard on the outsiders who do the pioneering work, and their stories can be excessively romanticized. Producers and consumers of popular entertainments love a good tale of an outsider who nobly suffers to bring the world something new. I can't claim to be in this dramatized company because my own career has never been mortally threatened by my differences with the mainstream of the medical profession. The clinical results of my methods have been heartily welcomed by patients, and this is what counts. When word spread that my placenta-based treatments were having unusual success in helping patients who were up against agonizing pregnancy problems, my practice flourished. My methods haven't caused me to be prevented from practicing medicine; I haven't been brought up before any professional inquisition; no professional body has ever accused me of misconduct. Lawsuits against medical practices are so common that they must include costly litigation insurance in their business overheads. Many doctors become quite familiar with courts and lawyers as a part of the routine conduct of their work. To my great happiness, I've managed to steer unusually clear of legal battles. On the contrary, I've received professional recognitions as an effective physician. I see all this as a testament to the fact that the lessons I've learned from my patients are ones that work.

Nevertheless, I'm known in my profession as a maverick because my treatment methods differ from those used by most maternal-fetal specialists, and while this hasn't led to any formal disputes between myself and other physicians, it's definitely affected my relationships with many. These things can be subtle. Will I be invited to a professional get-together? When certain doctors meet me in a hospital corridor, will they greet me and chat with me in the same friendly tone they've just used in conversing with some other physicians who happen to share their clinical philosophy? Cliques can shun in delicate but intensely meaningful ways without doing anything clearly identifiable as victimization. Quite a few physicians have expressed their disapproval of my methods in unspoken but eloquent ways, keeping their professional distance. This has caused me no sleepless nights, though. In fact, I can hardly imagine anyone being more fulfilled by work than I am. I've felt overwhelming joy as mother after mother, year after year, has given birth to a healthy baby after being led to believe it would never happen. I'm also often gratified to come across appreciative colleagues who agree with my treatment approaches even if only privately. And yet it's also been personally transforming for me, both sad and in a way strangely liberating, to learn that, if I wanted to heal damaged pregnancies as well as I could, I'd have to be prepared to break away from that medical mainstream which once, as a young doctor, I'd regarded as virtually infallible in its wisdom. This break has revolved around my clinical finding, again and again, that the initial 12 weeks of pregnancy contain the keys to a healthy placenta.

~

Let's pause here for another summing-up. The placenta grows continually until birth, depending for this on blood supplied by two circulation systems, the mother's and the baby's. These systems can be impaired by clotting problems affecting the placenta at different times and in ways that vary from patient to patient. This wide variation is fundamental in determining the right treatment. Not all patients respond alike to the same treatment. Mothers should be fully examined not later than the fifth week, or as soon as possible thereafter. Many doctors will tell you nothing can be done for your pregnancy in the initial three months but substantial clinical experience shows they're wrong. Evidence indicates that at least half of all first-trimester miscarriages involve chromosomally normal embryos. To save these babies, the placenta should be evaluated at five weeks, then every two weeks until around week 32; then weekly or even more often if needed. Doppler technology must be used to ensure acceptably low resistance in the uterine blood vessels. The higher the resistance, the less blood the placenta gets, and the resistance depends on how healthy the spiral artery remodeling has been; successful remodeling should have deprived them of their ability to constrict, so blood can flow freely into the placenta to ensure a well-nourished, properly developed fetus. The initial 12 weeks are critical time for this. A small placenta at 12 weeks means a growth-retarded baby. Contrary to the belief that we can do nothing for the baby in those early weeks, we can avoid such problems, with profound implications for the baby's health, if we catch the problems early enough in that crucial 12-week window.

We can also treat such patients helpfully after 12 weeks, but then it won't be an optimal pregnancy. The baby will be at risk of growth problems and prematurity because untreated development loss in the initial 12 weeks can't be reversed completely.

At whatever stage we start managing the pregnancy, the monitoring must serve not just to check for problems but also to find out whether a treatment is working. Instead of doctors saying vaguely, "Let's try this treatment and see how the pregnancy turns out," we can now map a treatment's effects week by week. In the 21st century, it's a doctor's responsibility to do this. Too much is at stake for mother and baby for this not to happen. Monitoring can also confirm whether the problem is getting worse, or being complicated by other problems, prompting the doctor to change the medication or its dosage or frequency, or to prescribe supplementary medication. Thus, if it emerges that a mother's clotting problems are caused by both immune-system and genetic problems, and LMWH doesn't work well enough on its own, another medication like a corticosteroid or an intralipid might be added to the treatment.

The effectiveness of intralipids has been a happy revelation in pregnancy care. This medication can make a huge difference for the outcomes of pregnancies with increased and abnormal Natural Killer cells, as we saw in the case of Miranda and her twins, where her fertility treatment had included intralipid infusions for NK cell issues. In line with the prevailing guidelines, you'll recall, her infusions were stopped by week 12 of the pregnancy, but between her 14th and 16th weeks, one twin's umbilical artery circulation and placenta weakened ominously, and after two more weeks fetal growth was stunted, with poor umbilical blood suggesting that the impaired baby had zero chance of normal health, with its survival in question. Worse, its sibling also faced severe impairment unless the problem twin was terminated. Miranda responded by asking for her treatment with steroids and intralipids to be resumed. Though it was unprecedented, her request was granted, and after two weeks the umbilical artery blood flow totally recovered. Both twins were eventually born healthy, showing that intralipids can work right until the 9th month.

Miranda's case also illustrated the importance of umbilical artery blood flow. We've seen that the less resistance in the umbilical artery, the more easily blood flows from baby to placenta. As the baby grows, a healthy placenta makes more supplementary blood vessels available to meet demand. If this doesn't happen, high umbilical artery resistance reduces blood flow between baby and placenta, which can cause the baby to grow poorly, be born prematurely, and perhaps die; this is why we should check the umbilical artery with Doppler ultrasound every two weeks.

It's also wise to monitor the development of the placental villi, those finger-like projections in the intervillous space which carry oxygen and food to the umbilical vein; the more villi, the better! As I explained earlier, having fewer villi opens the door to all kinds of fetal problems from poor growth to death, and persistent villi weakness is the first sign of placental failure, an invaluable early warning system. If the villi scream for help, urgent action is needed! Studies indicate that, by the time fetal umbilical-artery blood flow has weakened enough for Doppler ultrasound to detect it, almost 30% of the villi will already have deteriorated, so it's foolish to rely only on fetal umbilical-artery monitoring: your doctor must monitor those villi as well, to detect major problems and treat them long before 30% of the villi are damaged because that level of harm will leave even the most successful treatment unable to help the baby achieve its full potential. The amount of placental damage shapes the pregnancy's outcome. The evidence on this is terrifying, linking normal placentas (no clotting damage) with the best pregnancy outcomes (no pre-eclampsia; only some 3% of babies with growth problems; less than 8% prematurity), while linking placental clotting damage with incidences of preeclampsia at 9%, growth problems at over 15% and prematurity at 18½%. These bad outcomes happened not just with heavy clotting damage but any clotting damage. The amount of damage in these recorded cases did make a difference to the level of risk of prematurity, growth restriction, pre-eclampsia and possible fetal death, though. With lesions (areas of damaged tissue) exceeding about two inches (about five centimeters), the prematurity risk was four times greater than with normal placentas, the growth restriction risk 13 times greater, and the average baby weighed two pounds less than one with a normal placenta. With placental lesions smaller than five centimeters, average baby weight shifted toward 1½ pounds less than with a normal placenta. Over 30% of babies with the worst placentas were premature; over 38% had abnormal growth.

These devastating facts mean significantly increasing risk of fetal death and, for surviving babies, of illnesses in the long term. The two main contributors to the illness and death of babies, both unborn and newborn, are prematurity and growth failure. Of every 13 mothers with recorded lesions exceeding five centimeters, two lost their babies, i.e. a 15% fetal death rate, which is 15 to 30 times greater than the general population's, depending on how this population is defined. Thus, placental clotting problems must always be caught early enough and treated even if neither mother nor fetus is diagnosed with thrombophilia, and even if the mother's blood tests are normal. The placenta is the battleground of all clotting and anti-clotting factors. Medical science can't yet measure the many ways in which these factors interact with each other; there are too many and they're too complex. But we know enough to see and monitor the kind and extent of their effects, to administer effective treatment when the problems are caught early enough, and to adjust the treatment according to how rapidly placental lesions develop and how they respond to treatment. Clinical experience shows that if all goes well and the pregnancy reaches week 32, monitoring should occur weekly or more frequently depending on what we've learned about the placenta, fetal and uterine blood flow, and biophysical profile, or BPP, a composite fetal assessment including the amount of amniotic fluid (which, you may recall, fills the protective bag around the unborn baby) as well as the baby's movement, breathing and muscle tone. The baby must also be checked regularly for possible umbilical cord compression and for the rate of blood flow into the brain and in its descending aorta. Doppler must be used wherever appropriate. Blood flow in key arteries can alert us to serious problems before the baby itself is affected. Most doctors measure the baby's heart rate with the "non-stress test" (NST) which, as I've explained, my clinical experience indicates is ineffective. My clinical experience has been confirmed by several major randomized clinical trials that found NST to be worthless and potentially dangerous … and yet it remains the standard of care for decades! It should be replaced by Doppler.

Virtually everything I've talked about so far has arisen from the fact that every pregnancy is unique, and now I want to tell you about a case which illustrates this uniqueness in a very special way.

Chapter 22

RUTH'S STORY

As we've seen, the cervix is the opening between the uterus (womb) and the vagina. As I write this, Ruth's cervix has a cerclage, the stitch that a physician may apply to protect a fetus where the cervix is weak: the doctor sews the cervix closed to help keep the baby where it should be until birth. A cerclage in itself isn't unusual. It's routinely used in certain pregnancy conditions. However, at the time I am setting this down for you to read, Ruth isn't pregnant, although she has four healthy children. Why, then, is she walking around with a cerclage? Therein lies the tale.

Ruth's pregnancy experiences (six of them as of this writing) left her with a cervix as perforated as a Swiss cheese, but at the same time they show that a woman's body can exceed the boundaries of what appears to be possible. Ruth also understood that if her cerclage was removed, it would be very hard to re-sew her cervix tissues together again. Her decision to go about her everyday life with a cerclage meant that if she and her husband decided to have another baby she'd be ready for one of the pregnancy complications that she realized could arise. A cerclage isn't left in place indefinitely, though; usually two years or so is the limit. In theory it can be left in longer, but in reality many patients then fail to return to their doctor for 6-monthly cerclage checkups, either because they forget or because they become complacent, and this can lead to problems. At any rate, Ruth knew she'd have to see her obstetrician every six months for a cervical culture, an analysis of a sample of matter from the cervix to ensure that no infection was developing. (My clinical team has used cervical cultures successfully to help patients keep a cerclage safely in place even after they experienced many cerclage failures before coming to us. One of our cerclage patients not only had a full-term pregnancy but then had another, with twins. I haven't seen such an outcome documented elsewhere.)

Ruth's first pregnancy, at age 21, was full-term, textbook-normal, uneventful and yielded a healthy son. But her next pregnancy brought trouble, beginning with severe lower back pain and uncomfortable pelvic pressure. Her obstetrician's explanation, excessive weight gain, didn't satisfy her so Ruth found another doctor who referred her to me when her water suddenly broke at 26 weeks. I diagnosed her symptoms as very early signs of preterm labor, which usually go unnoticed. She was treated with magnesium (not by me but briefly by her obstetrician) to stop contractions, and antibiotics to prevent infection, and was hospitalized for a couple of weeks. Such a long hospitalization was unusual. Delivery commonly follows within about 24 hours of the water breaking but the aim now was to keep her pregnant. An ultrasound revealed placenta damage caused by clots and a baby that was small for its age. Ruth didn't want to stay in the hospital, preferring to go home and come in for frequent blood tests, screening for infection and weekly ultrasound examinations. This was (and still is) acceptable management as long as the amniotic fluid level remained adequate and the patient was capable of following instructions at home. However, after a few days Ruth started bleeding, most likely because of the unhealthy placenta along with umbilical cord compression caused by amniotic fluid loss. Then disaster struck: a sonogram showed that the baby had died. At that stage, a big question was: what had caused her placental damage? While genetic testing showed she had thrombophilia, this alone couldn't explain the degree of damage. Her husband Boris (who wasn't the father of her first child) was now tested too. It turned out he had three serious genetic mutations that can cause fetal thrombophilia if a baby inherits them. Based just on her blood tests, in the absence of evidence of placental damage, Ruth wouldn't automatically have been treated for thrombophilia, but, given Boris's results, she was put on anticoagulation treatment with enoxaparin sodium and aspirin as soon as she conceived for the third time. Around 16 weeks into this new pregnancy, a sonogram showed her cervix had deteriorated disturbingly, increasing the risk of pregnancy loss. She was hospitalized and her cervix was stitched. Things still didn't go well. She was in great pain and on a morphine drip. Urinating was difficult as the cerclage procedure had compressed the bladder openings of her ureters (two tubes leading from the kidneys). Her first baby's cesarean section and her bladder scars were hindering her cerclage, which was consequently removed. I prescribed bed rest, the non-steroidal anti-inflammatory drug indomethacin, the blood pressure medicine nifedipine, and close monitoring. At 38 weeks she had a healthy daughter, Alice.

Now that she was more informed about pregnancy management, Ruth decided she wasn't going to leave her next pregnancy to chance. Almost two years to the day after Alice's birth, she conceived again. She followed the same medication regime as before and again had a cerclage. This time things went well. Her daughter Chloe arrived after 37 weeks. Then, nine months later, she became pregnant again, and this time a new problem arose: she found she couldn't return to my clinic, which had managed her pregnancies with Alice and Chloe, because we happened at that time to be in a dispute with her health insurer. Hundreds of patients were affected. I'll summarize it here because it sheds light on how the health system fails pregnant mothers. In cases like Ruth's, my clinic requires mothers to be examined every two weeks. Following Chloe's birth, Ruth's insurers considered this examination regime unnecessary and refused to cover it, forcing her to seek care for her latest pregnancy from a perinatologist who complied with her insurers' rules omitting two-weekly examinations. Ruth's cervix suffered premature shortening and she went into preterm labor. She was again given a cerclage and a few days later, around 21 weeks, her amniotic sac broke, losing most of its fluid. Sadly, her new doctor had given her the cerclage without taking her placental problems into account, and treated her short cervix as intrinsically weak instead of as being inflamed by dead placental tissues. Evidence suggests this mistake is common and is why half of all cerclage procedures fail to protect the baby. It treats a symptom, cervical shortness, leaving the underlying problem, thrombotic placental damage, untreated so it gets worse; eventually the uterus can't cope and expels the baby.

Ruth would later recall her new doctor saying she could abort or wait for the baby to be expelled. On asking if the baby was still alive, and learning it was, she desperately called the obstetrician who'd originally referred her to me and was advised to return to my clinic. The insurance dispute was still under way, so we worked out a payment plan for her that enabled her to come back to us for treatment. By now, Ruth had learned enough about pregnancy to understand that a baby born at 24 weeks has a relatively low (54%) survival chance; of the survivors, 80% will probably have serious disorders like blindness, lung disease and cerebral palsy. The next day, an ambulance brought Ruth 75 miles from her home area to my clinic, where we found a grim situation: the baby's foot was ripping through her cerclage stitch. Labor had to be induced and the baby was lost. But the couple wanted more children, and as they were now convinced that a sensitivity to Ruth's placental history was vital, they asked my clinic to handle her next pregnancy. Fortunately, by then the insurance dispute had ended (more about this below) so I was able to continue to care for her. She quickly became pregnant again.

Around 28 weeks into this new pregnancy, the baby's heart reacted to the medicine indomethacin, causing narrowing of the ductus arteriosus, a major heart blood vessel. This is a known indomethacin side effect but usually doesn't occur until later in the pregnancy. She was taken off the drug and a plausible explanation emerged to account for the unexpectedly early manifestation of the side effect: at 28 weeks the baby was already as big as a normal 32-week baby (as a result of too much maternal weight gain from lack of activity and a bit too much food) and it is reasonable to suppose that this unusual size caused it to respond to the indomethacin as an older baby would. As always happens, the ductus arteriosus became normal again within 24 hours after we stopped indomethacin.

Ruth's fourth baby was a healthy son and I was very proud when she and Boris named him after me. And when I was writing this book, Ruth was still walking around with her cerclage, because despite the pregnancy problems she'd been through, she didn't rule out the prospect of having a fifth baby. Like me, she'd learned that pregnancy is so full of unpredictables that it seems almost a misnomer to say that it's about "expecting"; sometimes it seems to be even more about the unexpected.

Ruth's case illustrates significant shortcomings of conventional pregnancy care. While the placental problems that triggered her complications are far from unusual, they can have wholly unexpected results, especially in view of the relatively small attention that's commonly given to placental issues. The failure to see that inflammation from dead placental tissues lay behind Ruth's short-cervix condition (when she saw another specialist during the interruption of her care at my clinic due to the insurance dispute) illustrates a common tendency to ignore the placental origins of many pregnancy problems. Much cervical care is impaired by this flaw, which is complicated by the failure of most randomized clinical studies to document cerclage benefits. This failure encourages a climate of thought in which many influential physicians not only fail to recognize that something is wrong with cervical diagnoses that ignore the placenta, but even also conclude that cerclage itself should not be used. This error arguably contributes to thousands of premature births and many more complete pregnancy losses. Ruth's story also illustrates the important fact that fathers often hold the key to diagnosing and treating pregnancy complications. Yet, despite the instances of paternal testing that I've illustratively included in this book, the contributory and diagnostic role of fathers is so egregiously ignored in conventional pregnancy management that it's rare indeed for a father to be tested for thrombophilia during pregnancy, despite the common need for this to be done.

RUTH'S STORY

By the way, that dispute with the insurance company is long and intricate, but pregnant mothers facing potential pregnancy complications should know about the power that insurers have over pregnancy management, so I'll summarize it here. At the time, I was working with that insurance company in-network. When they decided to stop paying me for patient examinations which exceeded their arbitrary rule, I liaised with them for over six months to explain to them that, in addition to being medically essential for the patients and their babies, the examinations greatly served the insurance firm's financial interests by helping prevent medical problems in mothers as well as in babies who would need expensive care if they were born impaired. I presented clinical and financial evidence demonstrating that for every 1000 pregnancies that my clinic managed using our methods of close monitoring, we saved the insurer almost $26 million which they would otherwise have had to pay for the medical treatments that our methods made unnecessary. To my astonishment, they showed no interest in this. The reason for their indifference, I then discovered, was that health insurers buy reinsurance from other insurance companies, insuring themselves against the costs of their clients' catastrophes. If Ruth's baby was born at 26 weeks and spent eight weeks in the NICU (neonatal intensive care unit), costing hundreds of thousands of dollars, Ruth's insurers wouldn't have to pay this bill; the reinsurance company would pick up the tab. Thus, Ruth's possible catastrophes were of no interest to her insurers. They were interested only in her non-catastrophic visits to our clinic, because those were the ones they, and not the reinsurer, had to pay for. Bizarrely, it was in their financial interest to minimize Ruth's examinations at my clinic even if in so doing they increased her risk of catastrophes! It is with dismay and grief that I now know that providers of pregnancy care work in this immoral climate, which flatly contradicts what I regard as fundamental medical ethics. Physicians who cooperate with these callous corporate behemoths are helping to restrict patient access to care. What a mockery this makes of the Hippocratic oath that the public associates with doctors, and which requires physicians to do no harm or injustice to their patients.

This horrible sickness in our medical establishment was brought home to me further when an obstetrician working for one of the largest insurance companies called to tell me they'll no longer pay for fetal umbilical artery Doppler studies unless the baby's weight drops below the 10th percentile, i.e. requiring me to let babies suffer the maladies of the gravest degree of fetal growth retardation, with all its lifelong health impacts, before I can examine them properly in order to treat them precisely to try to prevent those very impacts. This is made all the more terrible when you consider that my expertise is supposed to be aimed at protecting these babies from losing even a few ounces of their growth potential. When I pointed out the insurance company's obstetrician what a travesty of medical ethics this was, she cleared her throat and in a solemn, authoritative tone informed me that her company's policy was consistent with the guidelines laid down by ACOG, the American College (formerly Congress) of Obstetricians and Gynecologists. This leads to the question: what are ACOG guidelines? The answer is that they are communications on clinical matters which are no more than a kind of CliffsNotes for obstetricians and gynecologists. They're not intended to offer detailed instructions on clinical care and are certainly not meant to be legally or medically binding on health care providers in any way. Essentially, they offer information for physicians to use at their discretion as the basis of a framework for clinical thinking. It is up to individual medical practitioners to decide how they interpret, apply, deviate from or enlarge upon the guidelines as they consider appropriate in light of their moral responsibilities, as they understand these, and in light of the needs of the patients for whom it's their duty to care. ACOG makes the limited and provisional nature of its guidelines very clear, by attaching to them disclaimers like "the information should not be construed as dictating an exclusive course of treatment or procedure to be followed," "this information is designed as an educational resource to aid clinicians in providing obstetric and gynecologic care, and use of this information is voluntary," "this information should not be considered as inclusive of all proper treatments or methods of care or as a statement of the standard of care. It is not intended to substitute for the independent professional judgment of the treating clinician. Variations in practice may be warranted when, in the reasonable judgment of the treating clinician, such course of action is indicated by the condition of the patient, limitations of available resources, or advances in knowledge or technology," and "publications may not reflect the most recent evidence."

I consider it to be a shocking abuse of these ACOG communications to cite them as excuses or pretexts to justify the insurance industry behavior I've described. Given this insurance industry culture, and the immense power that the industry wields over the medical services available to mothers and babies, that maternal mortality in the US has been on the rise since the early 1980s and is now three times that of the rest of the Organization for Economic Co-operation and Development (OECD), a community of nations producing most of the world's wealth. Over the same period, premature births in the US have risen from less than 8% in 1980 to almost 12½%, and in some states 14%, placing the US on par with the poorest countries. The US also has the highest infant mortality (death between the ages of one month and five years) in the OECD.[144] This is a remarkable and disgraceful comedown for an America which was once the world's gold standard for medical care. Because ACOG's guidelines are being cited to justify insurance practices which contribute to this mess, I believe ACOG has a responsibility to take action to rein in the insurance industry's abuse of the guidelines, and other medical organizations should join in such corrective action. But I believe this is unlikely to happen unless there is a sufficient public outcry, and this is something in which readers of this book can play a helpful role. I hope you will take to social media to make your voice heard in this connection. Until adequate action is taken, the ACOG guidelines will be an immense tombstone on the graves of all babies who have been sacrificed to callous and atrocious insurance industry policies.

You may wonder what happened to the baby about which the insurance company obstetrician called me to deny coverage for Doppler exams unless the baby's weight dropped under the 10th percentile. The baby's growth fell to below average between the 14th and 18th weeks, making it likely that without the Doppler exams that were being denied, and the detailed diagnosis and treatment that these exams would make possible, the baby would likely be growth-retarded around 26-28 weeks, a point at which it would be too late to prevent premature delivery and a high probability of serious health issues lasting into adulthood. Since I could not bring myself to let this happen, I took matters into my own hands and, without insurance support, I responded to the warning signs that the baby's placenta had already provided (which the insurers would not recognize) and adjusted the mother's treatment accordingly, waiving the payment that the insurers would have made if they had agreed to cover the necessary Doppler exams and related treatment. Within two weeks of treatment adjustment, the baby's growth stabilized. Because we caught this problem early, albeit without insurance support, growth then accelerated and reached a healthy level. But if we had complied with the insurers' inappropriate application of the ACOG guidelines, which were inapplicable to this case, the baby wouldn't have received treatment when needed but would have been classified as normal until it had suffered irreversible growth retardation. Only then would the insurance-compliant obstetricians have sounded the alarm… too late. Sadly, it's beyond the capability of my clinic to provide free services in this way to all the patients who need it. They'll receive the care they need only if and when public outrage causes politicians to change how the health insurance industry works.

To sum up: the insurance policies I've been talking about were the cause of a general dispute that my clinic was having with Ruth's insurers when she happened to need treatment, which was why her treatment by us was interrupted. Many other patients were also affected. My clinic's aim at that time was try to persuade the insurers to change their policies. The clinic had to hire expensive lawyers to help with this, and eventually we had to end those particular efforts to bring about an insurance change because we could no longer afford it, while the insurance company was so rich it could keep up the legal battle virtually endlessly. I came away from the experience with a deepened appreciation of the power of insurers, and, to this day, insurance companies continue to refuse to cover essential, life-saving medical care in cases like Ruth's, even though abundant clinical evidence exists to show convincingly that frequent, intensive, pre-emptive and proactive monitoring is medically necessary for such patients. And that battle was just one of many in an ongoing war. Not a month goes by without insurers trying to get out of paying for some part of the care I believe my patients need. It could be argued that I shouldn't be a physician if I'm unable to stomach this. But what about the mothers and babies who struggle to get essential care because insurers reject medical facts? As far as we know, three-quarters of all pregnancies fail, and 30% of pregnancies have outcomes including pre-eclampsia, growth problems, cerebral palsy, PROM (premature rupture of amniotic membranes), placenta abruptio, various genetic defects and prematurity, which causes 80% of all newborn deaths and sickness. You'd think that as part of our healthcare system medical insurers would want to do whatever they can to reduce these shockingly high rates of death and illness. But this doesn't seem to be the case. It is to our national shame that around 1980, no more than 8% of US pregnancies were premature, but that today it's 12½%, a more than 50% increase despite the stated goal of two US Government agencies, the National Institutes of Health and the Centers for Disease Control and Prevention, to reduce the figure to 5% by the year 2000. When that goal wasn't achieved, 2010 was aimed for. But that wasn't achieved either. The goalposts have since been moved to 2020, and I feel sure they'll be moved yet again to keep up with our healthcare system's consistent record of spectacular failure. And this is happening in the 21st century, in the richest, allegedly most scientifically advanced country in the world. Pre-eclampsia continues to be a significant cause of death for mothers and babies, cases of diabetes in pregnancy have quadrupled and are increasing, growth retardation is up.

It's important to understand that this dire situation isn't due to a want of knowledge and technology. Our physiological, genetic and biochemical knowledge has been advancing hugely, and we now have plenty of information about placental warning signs that tell us when the health of a placenta (and therefore the success of the pregnancy) is headed the wrong way. It's on the level of health care policy that the medical establishment is failing in patient treatment and crucial steps to prevent disease. There are no excuses for this miserable failure, which is due plainly and simply to the medical establishment's persistent refusal to respond to placental warning signs and act on them to stop pregnancy disorders at the outset, instead of letting them happen and then struggling to cure them, commonly too late. If doctors fail to prevent a pregnancy complication, there's generally a strong likelihood that the pregnancy will have to be interrupted. For example, if a mother develops pre-eclampsia at 27 weeks, the baby will likely be delivered prematurely and the placenta removed to save the mother's life. And as I've explained, preterm birth afflicts a baby with lifelong health consequences.

We've seen in earlier pages that one of the commonest mistakes in pregnancy care is to see events in isolation, as if they're unrelated. This seriously obstructs the effective prevention of complications, because mother, placenta and baby aren't isolated, unrelated phenomena: they form a closely interwoven organic whole. In recent decades, several so-called "silver bullet" tools have emerged to help doctors determine who will develop pre-eclampsia, but these have had questionable effectiveness, largely because so many doctors see preeclampsia as a self-contained phenomenon rather than as being rooted, as it is, in the earliest stage of pregnancy, when implantation issues create conditions leading to various immune-system, vascular and clotting problems. Failure to approach diagnosis and treatment of the disease in the light of this key fact is a major handicap blocking proper understanding and care of pre-eclampsia. Here's why: if the placenta isn't properly examined early enough, the physician, mother and baby are then at the mercy of the next signs that a patient is at increased risk to develop pre-eclampsia. But these signs show up only at 12 weeks, by which time the fuse of the pre-eclampsia bomb has already been lit. Once the fuse is lit and we know preeclampsia is on the way, we have no idea when it will strike. It can be any time after the twenty-second week. After it strikes, the only cure is removing the placenta. Clearly, then, what we have to do is look after the placenta early enough that the fuse isn't lit. Failing to do this is a pretty awful reflection on our medical establishment considering that eclampsia, the fatal end-stage of preeclampsia, was first described by Hippocrates, who lived over 2000 years ago.

By the way, preeclampsia's key cause, placental clotting, is also the common denominator linking all pregnancy complications and disasters: PROM (premature rupture of membranes),[145-147] growth restriction, placenta abruptio, preterm birth, cerebral palsy, and death of the baby. Given this, it's no surprise that anti-clotting care is the common treatment for these placenta-related problems. In a study by researchers unaffiliated with my clinic, mothers with a 30% risk of pre-eclampsia were given 40 milligrams of the anti-clotting medication LMWH daily throughout their pregnancy. Placenta-related problems decreased remarkably: in particular, pre-eclampsia dropped 74% compared with mothers who weren't treated in this way. Growth restriction fell 77%. For early severe pre-eclampsia cases, the drop was 88%; early intrauterine growth restriction fell 86%. And uterine artery resistance relaxed to a healthy degree over the course of the whole pregnancy for the treated mothers.[122] Most obstetricians have largely ignored these results, probably because they were published in the American Heart Association's journal Hypertension, which few obstetricians read. This is far from the only case where obstetricians haven't been keeping up with vital information because it's published in journals not aimed primarily at obstetricians. This is unjustifiable. Obstetricians should make it their business to keep up with information important to their professional responsibilities no matter where it's published. The above research findings, from independent researchers unrelated to my clinical team, are wholly consistent with our clinic's data. Our files document the history of patients who've been monitored fully from early pregnancy and treated with anti-clotting medication as considered necessary, and these files show that in such cases the incidence of early preeclampsia is almost zero, while mild late-onset preeclampsia happens in a little over ½% of cases. This represents a reduction of more than 95% compared with the general rate for the average pregnant woman. And our clinical records show an almost zero incidence of the early-onset severe form of preeclampsia. (According to the Preeclampsia Foundation, preeclampsia strikes 10 million women annually worldwide and about 76,000 pregnant women die every year from this and related hypertensive illnesses, which kill an estimated 500,000 babies a year.) These results, published in peer-reviewed medical journals, apply to singleton pregnancies. But the placenta-centered management that they reference works as well or even better with twins, triplets or more babies. The usual incidence of preeclampsia with twins is 25%. Our records show that the application of the methods described in this book result in an incidence of between 2% and 3%. The uterine arteries, which are affected by conditions like pre-eclampsia, are important not only to supply food and oxygen to the placenta and thus to the baby, but also to ensure that the cervix is strong enough to support the baby for nine months. If the supply of enriched, oxygenated blood to the uterus is poor (ischemia), dead cells accumulate in the placenta and the lining of the uterus (the decidua). The body doesn't like this accumulation of dead cells, so the immune system turns a squadron of white blood cells into macrophages, which we've met in earlier pages; these objects digest unwanted matter such as the sick and dead placental and decidual cells, and, as a by-product of this digestion, the molecules called cytokines (which we also came across before) are formed. These molecules jump on the collagen fibers out of which the cervix is woven, and break them down. Collagen is the same substance that cosmetic surgeons inject to make lips fuller and smooth out wrinkles. If the collagen fibers in the cervix are damaged by too many cytokines, the cervix can become so weak that the risk of preterm birth, and associated conditions like PROM, rises greatly. If PROM (premature rupture of membranes) occurs, the mother, the baby or both can develop infections like chorioamnionitis, which inflames the amniotic membranes and can cause fetal brain damage and death. This infection often shows only after the baby is in trouble. If serious infection spreads through the mother's body, she may die. Poor uterine blood supply can cause PROM in different ways. You see, the amniotic membranes protecting the baby get fed partly by the amniotic fluid but mainly by the blood vessels of the uterine lining. Ischemia starves these membranes so that they wither and eventually rupture. A blood clot can also tear them away from the uterus. These are all additional reasons why it's essential to do everything possible to maintain healthy placental circulation.

RUTH'S STORY

In the general population, PROM tends to strike some 8% of pregnancies before the start of labor.[148] The clinical methods described in this book can cut this rate to a little over $1/2$%, which is a 90% improvement.[107, 108] Since 30% of all premature births result from PROM occurring before week 37, and more than 4 million live babies are born in the US every year, it follows that, if all doctors adopt these methods, around 120,000 of these babies will be born healthier and more safely! Your baby could be one of them. Because of this, it's important for us to dwell a little longer on the subject of health insurance and the financial challenges of pregnancy complication.

Chapter 23

THE PRICE OF AN IMPAIRED PLACENTA

On average, a preterm baby in New York today may cost patients, insurers and taxpayers up to half a million dollars or even more, from birth to the time the baby goes home. Of course, this financial cost is less important than the fact that prematurity is the top cause of newborn deaths. But it's important also to grasp that the staggering financial implications of this failure extend far into the lives of babies who survive. Fetal growth retardation (such babies are called "small for gestational age") caused by abnormal placental clotting has been increasing, now afflicts 8% to 9% of all pregnancies and is the main and sometimes only cause of many adult diseases. Also, mothers with placental problems are likelier to develop heart and circulation problems later in their lives. Patients (mothers and babies alike) who've experienced placental syndrome are likelier to die from heart and blood vessel diseases in midlife and beyond if they're not treated in time. Now, most researchers agree that placental syndrome conditions are caused by placental weakness associated with clotting problems, but they disagree as to whether these conditions can be prevented. Why? Well, I've already talked about how doctors can choose to reject evidence and prefer familiar ideas to unfamiliar ones. It's difficult for me to see any other reason than this for the disagreement, given the mass of evidence that compellingly tells us placental syndrome conditions can be prevented and even completely eliminated for most pregnant women. In patients with poor pregnancy histories, it's preferable for the pregnancy to be planned and for the mother to be treated from conception if not sooner. This is medically achievable and will usually assure a normal, undisturbed placental development which in turn will promote healthy fetal development, substantially reducing the chances of all serious adverse outcomes. As Ruth's case illustrates, though, health insurers are very reluctant to pay for these life-saving, health-promoting, illness-preventing measures.

My experience in high-risk pregnancy care has led me to see insurers as middlemen who syphon an enormous amount of money out of our national health care budget while impeding the prevention of disease, thereby increasing overall costs tremendously. In recent decades, the administrative costs of healthcare have been rising four times faster than physician-related costs. The successful pregnancy management methods I've been describing to you can save the US an enormous amount of money by enabling us to prevent expensive illnesses, which is generally much cheaper than curing them. Our ability to act on this principle may determine whether in future we'll have an effective health services system at all, especially when you consider that prematurity is one of our costliest health care issues. Here are some illustrative numbers based on my analysis of a sample of 1000 of my high-risk patient files. Ongoing analysis of other patients consistently supports these figures. By treating these

1000 patients with the placenta-based methods described in this book, the following pregnancy disorders, which were highly likely without treatment, were prevented: 132 cases of pre-eclampsia which would have cost at least $20,000 each; 18 cases of placenta abruptio which would have cost at least $20,000 each; 82 cases of PROM which would have cost at least $30,000 each; 215 cases of preterm delivery which would have cost at least $100,000 each; 71 cases of preterm hospital admission which would have cost at least $20,000 each. This totals $28,380,000 (twenty-eight million, three hundred and eighty thousand dollars) that no one had to spend because illnesses were prevented instead of waiting for them to happen and then curing them. The above 1000-case sample also shows that placenta-based treatment saved 250 babies whose lives would very likely have been lost without the treatment. While it's impossible to put a financial value on these lives, the above financial estimates aren't guesses. They're based on treatment cost estimates published in obstetric journals and are conservative, since, I explained earlier, wherever I estimate medical costs, I base my estimates on cost data from US states where prices tend to be on the low side. I believe my figures are much more reliable than most health cost analyses published today, which usually come not directly from doctors but from the administrative databanks of bodies like cooperative health organizations ("managed care organizations"), whose accounting systems, in my opinion, tend to record costs relatively crudely, glossing over important distinctions between types and severity of illnesses and even between types of doctor and treatment.[149] Many health cost analyses also use numbers from institutions whose departments maintain records in isolation from each other without properly reflecting the total cost of a patient who uses the facilities of more than one department. Significant outpatient costs are also often omitted. Similar limitations affect insurance data systems. Expense records are complicated further when families have more than one insurer. All this makes it hard to see the real costs of prematurity. In one case where complete expenses were captured for a premature delivery in New York, the baby's 41 days of intensive care treatment racked up a total bill of $1,200,000. This excludes the lifelong costs that will be incurred by the baby's severe handicaps resulting from prematurity. All these expenses could have been avoided by sufficiently early monitoring and treatment: when this same mother later received the correct placenta-based preventive care, she went on to have two more healthy babies after full-term pregnancies.

Paradoxically, the healthcare industry is profit-driven and thus concerned to cut expenses, yet its desire to wait for people to get sick and require expensive cures, instead of preventing sickness, is inefficient and wasteful. This paradox stems from a failure to understand that effective health care requires long-term thinking, which is undermined by policies which prioritize the short term. Insurance organizations promote themselves as being concerned with wise, long-term planning, yet in my experience their chief question tends to be *How much money can we save quickly?* rather than *How much money can we save in the longer term if we spend some more short-term money to prevent sickness?* This short-sighted approach, focusing less on long-term patient health than on the next quarter's earnings that will decide executives' bonuses, is surely the worst way to run the healthcare industry or our society. It disregards the future by placing as many obstacles as possible in the way of legitimate, clinically appropriate services and diagnostic testing. In this way, the insurance industry transfers financial assets from patients and health care facilities to industry executives in the form of big salaries and bonuses. My experience has led me to see this industry as a kind of parasite, with quality of health care being the last thing on its collective mind. The healthcare industry itself is ill. Curing it will take the cooperation of patients, doctors, politicians and health care leaders who genuinely care about public health. Until a cure comes about, it will continue to be unnecessarily hard for mothers and babies (including the unborn) to receive affordable, effective, efficient, prevention-oriented health care. Although this is a book about pregnancy, not economics or public policy, the healthcare industry determines your access to pregnancy care, so I've included this information to inform and encourage you to speak out to your doctor as well as to your friends, via word of mouth, social media and in any other way you can, to demand the early care that you and your baby need and deserve.

Although the patient stories I've shared with you have highlighted the kinds of pregnancy problems that proper placental care can address, early placental monitoring isn't just for pregnancies which are already known to have problems. Even for a mother with no history of pregnancy complications, early placenta assessment can help find out if she's at risk. Which may be the case. Early testing with the right anti-clotting treatment can detect and reverse a problem that's manifesting itself for the first time in a mother with no prior signs of complication, setting her and her baby on the road to a healthy pregnancy in conditions that could otherwise lead to a bad outcome. It's therefore a mistake, in my opinion, to allow many apparently low-risk pregnancies to go without an ultrasound exam until 18 to 22 weeks, given the complete formation of half the placenta's blood vessels by the 12th week, at which time it's too late to correct developmental damage to those vessels. In such cases, intense anti-clotting treatment for the rest of the pregnancy may still help the baby, but by that stage we have to live with the damage and work around it as best as we can. This harks back to the myth that first-trimester problems end when the calendar says the trimester is over. On the contrary, it's then that the undetected and untreated first trimester problems start showing their effects and reducing the likelihood of a successful pregnancy.

If placental problems are detected too late to reverse their effects, that will not make it futile to explore treatment options. Even when damage occurs, it may still be possible to manage its effects in the baby's interest. Here again, timing is crucial. If treatment begins before the damage becomes too entrenched. it's possible to reduce the 30% probability of preeclampsia superimposed on chronic hypertension by 90%, as well as to reduce the risk of first-time early severe preeclampsia by 98%, placenta abruptio by 66%, insufficiency of amniotic fluid (oligohydramnios) by 74%, preterm PROM (premature rupture of membranes) by 94%, preterm delivery by 80%, pregnancy loss by 86%, low birth weight by 82%, and preterm admission to hospital by 94%, while also protecting the baby 100% from fetal death due to placental insufficiency. This is all good news.[107, 108] It shows how far we've come in amassing clinical knowledge of how to save pregnancies despite the vastness of what we still don't know. And talking about this gap between what we know and don't know brings me to one of the biggest prematurity fears: the price that parents and baby have to pay when placental impairment damages the baby's brain development.

In the 19th century, a British doctor, William Little, suggested cerebral palsy was caused when a baby received insufficient oxygen during birth.[150] Today we know that birth asphyxia (lack of oxygen) plays a role in only a small percentage of cases of cerebral palsy, which is mostly caused by other problems. Most neurological disorders afflicting newborn babies are wrongly blamed on obstetric mismanagement at birth. This mistake has affected pregnancy care significantly and tragically. An unborn baby's brain grows most in the last three months of pregnancy, during which time it can be easily damaged by placental weakness, but most brain development problems aren't caused by insufficient oxygen either at birth or in the few weeks before birth. While the issue is controversial, extensive clinical experience indicates that popular views on fetal brain injury further illustrate the tendency to see pregnancy events in isolation instead of as parts of complex processes unfolding over time. There's a general failure to appreciate the complexity of the womb and what happens in it. For instance, when Dr Little studied children with cerebral palsy and found that many of them had a history of birth injury or birth asphyxia, the problem with his studies was that he studied only children who had cerebral palsy. He didn't study all the children who'd experienced birth injury or birth asphyxia but never developed cerebral palsy. These children are highly relevant to understanding how cerebral palsy and other brain disorders can be prevented. You'd think that, as information became increasingly available in the 20th century, the subject would have become clearer, yet it became more confused. In recent decades, obstetricians have been using tools like electronic fetal heart monitoring to prevent asphyxia from causing fetal brain injury. To call the results of these efforts disappointing is an understatement.

    Let's look at a few facts about the brain. To begin with, it's pretty small for such a complicated organ. The average adult brain weighs about three pounds, which is around 2% of the weight of a 150-pound person. But blood flow in the brain is about 750 milliliters a minute, which is some 15% of the body's blood flow. This means your brain uses almost seven times more blood, in proportion to its weight, than the rest of your body. To understand the importance of the brain's blood flow, consider this. I'm sure that at some point in your life someone has told you not to go swimming with a full stomach. This is not only good advice but can help you understand the importance of the brain's high blood flow. You see, when your stomach is full, your gastrointestinal system needs more blood to digest your food. This leaves less blood for your brain. If you immediately go swimming after eating a substantial meal, the blood supply to your brain is then reduced even further because the muscles you use for swimming also need blood. So you could end up with so little blood in your brain that you pass out and drown. This illustrates how sensitive the brain is to its oxygen supply. And if the adult brain is so sensitive, imagine how vulnerable a fetal brain must be.

Reduction in the brain's blood flow can be slow and gradual, or intense and quick (acute). Acute reduction in fetuses can result from an accident or an ongoing health problem. For example, if anything restricts the mother's breathing, the resulting oxygen shortage can cause the baby to die or suffer brain damage. Other causes of fatal oxygen loss include placenta abruptio and an umbilical cord accident. But the commonest cause is chronic placental insufficiency arising from gradual placental damage over time.

You'll remember that in Mary's case, we talked about the phenomenon of brain sparing, which protects the brain from oxygen-deprivation damage.[151, 152] Amazingly, fetuses have mechanisms capable of measuring the amount of oxygen in the blood, and they can adapt to compensate if chronic placental damage causes significant oxygen deprivation. They do this by changing the way their genetic programming expresses itself. Their circulatory system reorganizes its oxygen distribution so as to give priority to the brain, heart and adrenal glands. The blood vessels that deliver oxygen to these organs dilate to give them more blood, while the blood vessels that deliver to the rest of the body constrict to limit the amount of blood they carry. While these protective processes are remarkable, however, the best guarantee of healthy fetal brain development is a healthy mother. The weaker the mother's cardiovascular (heart and blood vessel) system, the higher the risk of placenta problems. Here are some of the cardiovascular weaknesses that can cause problems for the placenta (and thus the baby): age (the older the mother, the bigger the risk of cardiovascular problems), diabetes, kidney problems, chronic hypertension, poor weight before pregnancy (maternal weight gain during pregnancy is important for normal fetal growth but your weight before conception is even more important; low weight often indicates malnutrition, the occurrence of which in the critical first 24 weeks will obstruct placental growth severely), poor maternal weight gain after conception (a pregnant woman should gain, on average, 20 to 25 pounds during pregnancy, assuming she was at ideal body weight at conception; if she wasn't, she must gain enough to reach her ideal weight and then the additional 20 to 25 pounds: poor maternal weight will raise your baby's risk of pediatric and adult diseases in addition to the immediate risk of brain damage), heart and circulation disease (pregnancy increases the demands on a mother's cardiovascular function 50% for a single baby and 75% for twins; a compromised cardiovascular system can't handle the load and this can cause growth failure and/or brain damage); lung disease (your lung health is very important to your baby because your lungs provide all your baby's oxygen and expel all its carbon dioxide: any problem in your lungs can reduce your baby's oxygen, causing growth failure and/or brain damage; when a patient of mine became infected from a ruptured appendix and developed a lung illness called Adult Respiratory Distress Syndrome, or ARDS, she was in a critical condition for a week, breathing with the help of a respirator, and her baby didn't grow at all for two weeks.)

I now come to a chemical you need to know about because of its importance in the brain: serotonin. This chemical is a neurotransmitter, meaning it travels between nerves, helping them communicate. Low serotonin causes depression, while the drug cocaine increases the serotonin level and creates the "high" that cocaine users feel. But serotonin doesn't only create highs and lows of mood; it also regulates the structural development of the brain in the first six months of pregnancy. Because serotonin has this key role, it's produced by the placenta itself. There's good evidence that serotonin also influences the number of nerve cells in the vital area of the brain called the cortex, as well as the positions of these cells and how they wire up to other parts of the brain. So if the placenta becomes too weak to produce serotonin properly, this could obstruct early development of the cortex. If for any reason the placenta fails to produce enough serotonin, the baby's brain won't develop properly. We've only just begun to study what this means.[153, 154] The results could revolutionize the way we think about fetal brain damage and adult psychiatric conditions. For now this information further explains why your early placental health is so important not only for the pregnancy but for your baby's whole future life. While most cases of fetal brain damage were blamed for years on physical blunders that a doctor was assumed to have committed during the birth process, current information suggests that the real culprit is arguably an even worse blunder: the failure to appreciate how brain development problems, like so many others, have their roots in very early placental weakness, and in other placenta-related issues.

To produce serotonin the placenta first absorbs another chemical, tryptophan, from the mother's blood in the intervillous space. The placenta then converts the tryptophan to another chemical, which in turn is then converted into serotonin. Thus, if a mother doesn't eat enough foods containing tryptophan, this can promote conditions which obstruct the baby's brain development. My case files show a disturbing number of mothers with low-normal and below-normal tryptophan levels which, evidence suggests, can contribute to brain damage and later neurological and psychiatric disorders. And the ill effects of a tryptophan-poor diet can be magnified many times if the placenta has other development problems in addition to tryptophan insufficiency.

Some researchers believe the placenta has ways of regulating tryptophan levels to protect fetal brain growth, but there's not much convincing evidence of this. Available data do indicate (a) that doctors aren't currently monitoring tryptophan levels as they should, and (b) that this mistake stems from the obstetric profession's tendency to be quick to blame the placenta but to do nothing to identify a poorly functioning placenta early enough to treat it optimally. This behavior flows from the myth that nothing can be done to heal a malfunctioning placenta, which in turn harks back to that tendency to see pregnancy disorders as separate events which are somehow unrelated to the overall pregnancy process. Obstetricians' ability to see the diagnostic links between diverse pregnancy disorders has been profoundly damaged by this fragmentary vision. For example, seeing intrauterine growth retardation as something completely different from preterm labor, which in turn is seen as something unrelated to pre-eclampsia, is wrong, while cerebral palsy further illustrates the "isolated pregnancy disorder" mindset. As I've explained, the medical profession's sad failure to take adequate steps to prevent cerebral palsy has resulted largely from the erroneous tendency to associate it excessively or even exclusively with one event, fetal asphyxia caused by birth injury during delivery. Despite years of efforts to reduce the incidence of this kind of birth damage, the incidence of cerebral palsy remains stubbornly stable, and the reason for this is that the placental origin of much, if not most, cerebral palsy, as well as other neurological and psychiatric disorders, has been grossly overlooked. Compelling evidence indicates that the placenta's capacity or incapacity to produce the neurotransmitter serotonin is connected with the developmental programming of childhood and adult-onset mental illnesses. Genetic studies in mice suggest that disruption of serotonin activity before and after birth is associated with long-term behavioral abnormalities like increased anxiety in adulthood.[155, 156] (Earlier I warned against overestimating the human applicability of what we learn from mice and other animals, but I don't recommend ignoring such evidence either.) And it's interesting to note that commonly prescribed antidepressant medications are known to interact with serotonin.

Thinking about serotonin has progressed slowly. Only in the eight years or so preceding the publication of this book has it become understood that fetal serotonin in the first 24 weeks comes from the placenta, which synthesizes it from maternal tryptophan. A small amount also comes from the fetus. On the other hand, the long-held assumption that serotonin came only from the mother was supported by little if any empirical evidence.

This is one of many examples of how, if a respectable scientist makes a wholly unsupported assumption, the scientist's authority can promote its acceptance and perpetuation in the absence of evidence. But we know now that, as serotonin is instrumental to the early development of nerve networks in a baby's brain, reduced availability of it at this early stage can disrupt the growth of vital networks, contributing to defective intelligence, learning disabilities, depression, anxiety, autism, bipolar disorders and even schizophrenia.

So what can you do about all this? In addition to speaking out on this subject to your doctor, as well as to all your friends and family via social media and any other means, you can ensure not only that you receive the early placental screening and monitoring that you need, and any early treatment that you need, but also that you consume enough tryptophan to meet your baby's needs. You need to bear in mind early on in your pregnancy that a malnourished mother is likely to have low levels of tryptophan and also a small placenta, and that the combination of these two problems can curtail the placenta's production of serotonin, thus harming the brain development features that serotonin promotes. Tryptophan is present in many foods including seafood, meats and vegetables, so a well-chosen, healthy diet can ensure an adequate tryptophan supply, but how many people customarily follow a healthy diet? This isn't relevant just to your tryptophan intake, either. Your diet affects your pregnancy in many ways.

It's true that after they conceive, many mothers do try to

eat more responsibly, but the foods you ate in the months and years before pregnancy can continue to affect you during your pregnancy. Highly processed foods are common in the average American diet. Food processing adds hundreds of chemicals to our daily foods, while chemicals also enter the food chain during the production of so-called "natural" foods. Data indicate that some 70,000 chemicals are used in farming, meat production and preservation, and food refining and packaging with many lacking any testing for short-term or (even worse) long-term safety. A study by the Environmental Working Group, a non-profit consumer protection organization, tested fetal umbilical cord blood for 300 common chemicals of this kind and found 285 present.[157] What's more, women who don't eat healthy whole foods, but rely primarily on highly processed foods, are likely to lack enough essential minerals, amino acids, fatty acids, vitamins and antioxidants. Such deficiencies can interfere with normal fetal development in many ways, and women who eat mostly processed foods and very few unprocessed vegetables are very likely to run low on tryptophan. My website http://www.kofinasperinatal.org provides dietary information, including the tryptophan and glycemic content of various foods, to help you eat wisely during pregnancy.

Not every placental weakness is related to pre-existing problems with the mother's health, dietary or otherwise. For example, as far as we know, the placenta's position is random and has nothing to do with maternal pre-pregnancy habits or health. Remember, the placenta starts forming around six to eight days after conception, after the embryo implants itself in the uterine lining and starts the cellular invasion that leads to the remodeling of the spiral arteries. The placenta's location will depend on the embryo's: it may form at the top of the uterus or at the bottom, front, back, right side or left side. About half of all placentas grow in a more or less central position in the uterus, while half grow on the right or left side. Since the placenta's location can affect its blood supply, it's not surprising that studies confirm that when unilateral (off to one side) placenta's mean increased risk of poor fetal growth and pre-eclampsia. My files show some 30% of unilateral placentas as being associated with growth-retarded babies and/or pre-eclampsia, with the two uterine arteries, on the left and right of the uterus, seeming to lack proper connections, reducing placental blood flow. (One uterine artery alone can't supply all the nutrients the fetus needs, and the more relaxed an artery is, the easier the flow of blood.) The placental distribution of the hormone progesterone is also influenced by the placenta's position. A concentration of this chemical in tissues under and around the placenta helps keep the nearby uterine muscle fibers relaxed. Evidence indicates that, within that zone, the farther one goes from the placenta the less progesterone the tissues contain, so that the uterine muscle fibers in more distant areas are more tense and irritable, with greater tendency to constrict the uterus blood vessels. Such constriction reduces blood flow to the placenta even during the weak, normal contractions that all women experience during the entire pregnancy ("Braxton-Hicks contractions"). The arteries farther from the progesterone-protected placenta are in turn likelier to have restricted flow, reducing their ability to deliver food-and-oxygen-enriched blood to the placenta and the baby.

You may well ask: since the uterus contracts anyway during labor, why isn't the baby damaged by those contractions? Good question. In fact, the uterus contracts not only during labor (when the contractions are especially strong) but periodically throughout the pregnancy. It's not good for these pre-labor contractions to be too powerful, so while progesterone doesn't do away with them, it has an important job of keeping them at a moderate level, and it does this by relaxing the uterus muscle as I've described. Also, we saw earlier that when the spiral arteries under the placenta are remodeled, part of their remodeling consists of a loosening or relaxing effect, reducing their blood pressure to zero as the muscular wall of each spiral artery is destroyed and replaced by placental cells which are unable to contract. However, these very same arteries can be confidently relied on to deliver blood during labor, since no matter what contractions happen, these arteries can't be constricted. This arrangement protects the baby very well, as long as the placenta itself is big enough and healthy enough. The key fact here is that the spiral-artery protective mechanism is designed to function best when all placental conditions are working at their best. If the placenta isn't healthy enough in any respect, the protective mechanisms fall short and the baby will develop oxygen deprivation. In the worse cases, the baby may develop brain damage or die. Which brings me back to the unilateral placenta, and the fact that a placenta that grows off to one side is disadvantaged, not necessarily to a fatal extent but certainly to a serious one. If unilaterality happens to coincide with other placental weaknesses, the combined results can be very bad.

Although the determination of the placenta's location is currently understood to be random (a matter of chance), research is continuing and may reveal that it's affected by maternal health conditions that we can identify in advance, possibly enabling us in future to help every placenta grow in the best possible location. But for now, what matters to you and your pregnancy is that we know that unilaterality significantly increases the risk of pregnancy complications, and since steps can be taken to compensate for the problem if we learn about it in good time, this is yet another reason why your placenta should be assessed early. If unilateral development is detected, both main uterine arteries must be immediately evaluated by Doppler. If both uterine arteries have normal blood flow, the pregnancy will proceed normally. If the uterine arteries are compromised, such as by only one being normal (which happens in 30% of patients with unilateral placentas), the pregnancy will be at increased risk for fetal growth failure and pre-eclampsia and you must have a Doppler exam every two weeks to check fetal growth and oxygenation. This won't improve the placenta but it will help your doctor to protect your baby from brain damage and even death.

Chapter 24

THE ANATOMY OF A TEST

I've spoken a good deal about early exams and effective medical tests, but what exactly is an effective test? As with so much in medicine, the answer isn't necessarily what you might think. All tests aren't equal in value, so you need to understand what kind of testing will help you have a healthy baby. When science first began studying how the placenta works, doctors were mainly concerned with saving lives, and it was only in the second half of the 20th century that obstetricians began focusing not just on saving lives but also on helping babies develop as healthily as possible in the womb. After it became known that the placenta produces important hormones (chemicals that regulate health), tests were developed to enable doctors to measure the levels of hormones in women's urine, blood and saliva. The results were used to assess the health of both placenta and baby. However, although some later tests for placental proteins and hormones turned out to be helpful in detecting genetic defects like Down syndrome, as well as increased risks of placental weakness and fetal complications after the first three months of pregnancy, most of those 20th-century tests proved to be inconsistent and inaccurate, and today most have been abandoned completely in favor of another way to assess a baby's well-being: monitoring its heart rate.

Until 1958, we could hear a baby's heartbeat only via an obstetrical fetoscope, a device similar to a stethoscope. A midwife or nurse listened to the fetal heartbeat immediately after a contraction during labor. If the heartbeat sounded normal, labor was allowed to proceed. If the heart rate dropped, the baby was immediately delivered, vaginally (with vacuum extraction or forceps) or by cesarean section. (Such methods are terribly inadequate and don't reduce the risk of fetal death or severe damage.) Then, in 1958, Dr Edward H Hon designed the Doppler device that could record the fetal heartbeat, enabling doctors to identify potentially fatal problems in time to save the baby from death or brain injury. There are two kinds of fetal heart rate monitoring. One is the CST (contraction stress test), done in the final stages of pregnancy; there the heart rate is measured while uterine contractions are induced, to give the doctor an idea of how well the baby will cope with the stressful contractions of childbirth. The other test, which I've mentioned elsewhere in this book, is the NST (non-stress test), which involves continuous monitoring of the heart rate without contraction inducement. Let's look at each of these two tests. The CST doesn't really measure the baby's well-being: it just measures a specific response to artificially induced contractions at the time of the test. If the CST indicates that the baby struggles to cope with these artificial contractions, it doesn't necessarily mean a cesarean is necessary. The trouble is that most of these babies end up delivered by cesarean anyway. Many studies indicate that electronic fetal monitoring during labor might encourage unnecessary cesareans, including ones carried out in emergency conditions that can harm both mother and baby. The CST not only doesn't help babies, but it might even make birth less safe for baby and mother by leading doctors to perform the needless cesareans. Even more alarming is that doctors started using these tests without any studies indicating that there was a good reason to do so. So much for the CST. But how about the NST? That too presents a problem.

Despite the long use of NST monitoring, its value is controversial. While some studies support it, others suggest that its use has no effect on the number of deaths and brain injuries. A study published in the prestigious New England Journal of Medicine examined 34,000 pregnancies and found that whether fetal heart monitoring was continuous or intermittent made no difference at all to the pregnancy's outcome.[106] An analysis by the Cochrane Collaboration Group (which studies research results), published in 2008, assessed the results of 12 studies involving some 37,000 pregnancies and found that whether babies' heart rates were monitored or not made no discernible major difference to pregnancy outcomes.[158] The rate of fetal deaths, newborn deaths, cerebral palsy and other problems was much the same whether heart rate monitoring was done or not. Monitored fetuses had fewer fits, but the same rate of long-term neurological problems as unmonitored ones. In summary, there's no compelling evidence to show that the NST prevents any fetal death, cerebral palsy or other bad pregnancy outcome. Quite the opposite; on the contrary, in many studies up to 95% of fetal problems identified by NST monitoring turned out to be false results, serving only to scare the patient and her doctor and push them to take actions that were usually risky to both mother and baby.[159] Even worse is that in cases when NST use does manage to identify real problems, about half of those babies will already be too damaged to do anything about it. Two studies of babies who were smaller than they should have been (meaning they had experienced placental insufficiency), nearly half of them showed retarded development by the age of ten despite their NST results having been problematic. The NST is supposed to prevent such problems, but in this large number of cases it did not. This shows that by the time the NST is able to register an accurately positive result, the damage has been done. The test is therefore not only worthless but also dangerous because it provides a false sense of security even as the baby is being damaged. Children damaged in this way have a very high probability of being handicapped for the rest of their lives. So as a test to prevent fetal damage, the NST isn't much good. Yet the use of this test is currently the prevailing obstetric practice — the standard of care — in the face of solid evidence showing that this makes little sense. This goes back to my argument that doctors use many methods not because they're supported by evidence, but just because they've grown used to them. Change is hard: it calls for effort, it's inconvenient and sometimes quite painful. These are things no one wants, certainly. On the other hand, its human lives we're talking about. What's more, mistaken NST use doesn't just impact how obstetricians manage their patients' pregnancy care. It also obstructs the use of our precious research resources. Instead of trying to blaze new research paths that might show us better ways to protect babies, much research activity wastefully continues to cling to the NST, trying to rescue this kind of testing. An example of this effort to retain NST use is a device called a vibroacoustic stimulator, which is based on the idea that if the NST shows the baby's heart rate is abnormal, this might be because the baby is asleep. The vibroacoustic stimulator is supposed to awaken the baby to obtain a better test result. It does this with a noise as penetrating as that of a landing airplane. Apart from the ethics of subjecting an unborn baby to such a sonic assault, this is made questionable by the fact that, if the baby is sick, such a noise attack could force it to present an artificially elevated heart rate rather than the weak one whose accurate reading would reflect its real state of health. This amounts to masking a health problem instead of revealing it. To my mind this is poor medicine indeed.

Additionally, the NST is poor science, because deciding what its result means is highly subjective. Essentially it means whatever an individual doctor or researcher says it means. The result is a huge variety of criteria and interpretations whose results can conflict wildly. This is very remote from real science, which seeks objectivity rather than subjectivity, and uniformity rather than variation of result. Dressing it up impressively in the form of computer analysis, as has become fashionable, doesn't make it any better, because the computer simply spins out what a subjective human being has told it to do. And often the doctor will override the computer analysis with a personal interpretation, anyway. In 2006, Dr Michael Greene published an article in The New England Journal of Medicine titled *Obstetricians Still Await A Deus Ex Machina*.[160] His concluding paragraph says: "More than 30 years ago the new technology of electronic fetal heart-rate monitoring was introduced with the noble aspiration to eliminate cerebral palsy. We now find ourselves in the far less noble position of seeking new technology to mitigate the unintended and undesirable consequences of our last ineffective, but nonetheless persistent, technologic innovation."

As persistent and disturbing as it is, the NST fashion is by no means the only questionable practice that obstetricians have embraced. There's also the fashion of the Fetal Biophysical Profile (BPP). This test emerged out of studies done in the early 1980s in rural Canada, where many babies were dying of chronic placental insufficiency in the last few weeks of pregnancy. The BPP uses ultrasound to measure amniotic fluid volume as well as the baby's breathing, general body movement and certain specific movements ("tone"). The baby's "performance" in each area is measured in a number of points which are then added to make a total score. The NST is often incorporated as part of the BPP. Now, a healthy baby must of course be physically active, but breathing is surely a poor indicator of an unborn baby's vitality because, as I've explained elsewhere, fetuses don't really breathe. They do practice breathing motions, but even there they don't do it much. Accordingly, it's easy for an examination to miss fetal "breathing" and consequently give the baby a misleadingly bad score. On the other hand, some sicknesses can make a fetus mimic breathing motions excessively, which can also be misleading, because the BPP method tends to regard breathing movements generally as a good sign, so the more the baby is seen to "breathe," the better the BPP says it is ... even if the "breathing" is an expression of illness. Like electronic fetal heart rate monitoring, BPP was invented to prevent death in situations of chronic placental insufficiency, and when we look at it in this context it can, yes, be useful in certain high-risk pregnancies. However, it's not so good in measuring fetal well-being when an emergency situation isn't imminent. It's much like the NST in this respect: when the BPP is truly abnormal and the baby doesn't move, then the result is trivial because by then we have a real problem that it's probably too late to fix. In such a situation, the BPP may help the mother have a live baby instead of a dead one, but the baby almost certainly won't be healthy, and the BPP will have done nothing to help fix any health problem in time to avoid long-term damage to the baby.

    Then there's diabetes. Some years ago, experts at a highly respected institution published a report expressing surprise about four diabetic mothers whose babies died a day after a BPP test found them to be normal. Despite their distinguished status, these experts lacked basic understanding of how diabetes can give false BPP results. Diabetic mothers generally have higher levels of amniotic fluid than non-diabetic ones and their fetuses have increased breathing movements as well, because their excessive blood sugar produces too much carbon dioxide. Carbon dioxide stimulates the fetus's respiratory center, which in turn increases fetal breathing motions. But these phenomena signal sickness, and not (as the BPP interprets them) health! The NST can similarly misread diabetic pregnancies. And as I mentioned above, increased fetal breathing can give a misleading impression of healthy movement, both in its own right and by causing a fetal cardiac sinus condition which elevates heart rate variation (respiratory sinus arrhythmia), which NST testing interprets as a good thing. Which it is ... as long as the pregnancy is normal. But in diabetic pregnancies, increased heart rate variation can result from hypoxia (insufficient oxygen), making an ill fetus look healthy by BPP standards. On balance, BPP is a better test than NST alone, but as the above examples show, in many high-risk pregnancies it can produce false results, masking serious problems to an extent which could have life-threatening results. For example, in the case of fetal umbilical cord compression, the baby will breathe frequently due to hypoxia and may even be overly active before it dies. A BPP at such a time will tend to give a result that's not just falsely reassuring, but deadly.

If hypoxia is detected by Doppler, the baby should be delivered immediately to prevent brain damage. In the early 1980s, this technology improved significantly and was merged with new ultrasound systems, creating our best tool to assess placental and fetal health by directly measuring blood flow in a particular vein or artery, or by enabling us to calculate such flow based on the blood vessel's resistance to the blood. As I've explained elsewhere, Doppler's great and growing importance in managing complicated pregnancies makes it wise for every pregnant mother facing any degree of actual, or even possible, complication to have a basic understanding of how Doppler works. By bouncing sound waves off red blood cells as they rush into a blood vessel (either toward the placenta or away from it), picking up the bounced sound waves as they're reflected back from the moving red cells, and then analyzing these waves to calculate the speed with which the cells are moving, Doppler reveals the resistance in the blood vessel, enabling us in turn to calculate how much blood is being delivered, in which direction, and how effectively. Doppler has shown us that high resistance in placental vessels generally means poor placental health and increased risk of bad outcomes, including fetal growth restriction, insufficient amniotic fluid, cerebral palsy, development problems, the death of fetal bowel tissues (necrotizing enterocolitis), fetal death and newborn death. For placental and fetal health, the most important blood vessels that we measure with Doppler technology are the umbilical artery, which takes the baby's blood to the placenta, and the uterine artery, which takes the mother's blood to the placenta. Problems with either vessel system is bad, but the most shattering outcomes happen when both are sick. The timely use of Doppler technology is essential to avoid such events.

There are, broadly, three types of Doppler technology: CWD (continuous-wave Doppler), PWD (pulsed-wave Doppler), and CDI (color Doppler imaging). All show their results on a computer screen: in CWD and PWD, as a moving wave; in CDI, as a colored map of the blood vessels. Each type has its specific strengths (for instance, being able to tell blood vessels apart from each other accurately), and they can be used together to reinforce each other. Now, since what goes on in blood vessels is critically important for the placenta and thus for the baby's health during the pregnancy, at birth and after birth, the more we learn about blood pressure and blood flow inside the womb, the better it will be for your baby. For instance, increased resistance in the umbilical artery means increasing risk for fetal growth failure. I'm not talking about just one artery here. Even when we do talk about any major artery, that's just a convenient shorthand for what we're really talking about, which is always a vast system of blood vessels including the smaller vessels which lead off from every artery and form part of its total functioning. I've explained earlier how the umbilical artery, for instance, branches out into ever-smaller vessels in the placenta, like a tree whose trunk divides into main branches and then smaller ones, and finally into tiny twigs, eventually becoming microscopic capillaries in the placental villi. A normal placenta has an enormous number of villi and capillaries: the more blood vessel branches there are, the lower the resistance in the umbilical artery and the healthier the baby. The fewer the vessels, the smaller and weaker the baby. An important (but sadly little-known) study of umbilical artery resistance, aimed at helping growth-retarded fetuses improve enough to avoid irreparable damage or death, found that after taking low-dose aspirin for the rest of the pregnancy, mothers of such fetuses delivered babies that were half a pound to one pound heavier than the babies of untreated mothers.

Interestingly, as the number of Doppler studies has risen, so have the controversies. Most of these have not involved the umbilical artery as much the uterine artery, which is in some ways a more complicated vessel to study. For example, as the pregnant uterus expands into the upper abdominal cavity, the uterine artery actually changes in size and location, forming a moving target for ultrasound technicians and obstetricians, who can go crazy trying keep track of it. By comparison, the umbilical artery is easy to monitor. If its measurements stay too stable, this means placenta growth has stalled. If its resistance increases, this means placental vessels are constricted or aren't keeping pace with the baby's growth. Both are bad news. Like the umbilical artery, the uterine artery divides into hundreds of ever-smaller branches, thereby lowering blood-flow resistance. But the two arteries differ significantly in how their resistance relaxes during pregnancy. A healthy umbilical artery's resistance declines steadily until the pregnancy ends, while the uterine artery's resistance decline should be huge in the first three months of pregnancy, then slowing down and achieving maximum reduction around the 25th week; after that, only minimal changes occur toward the end of the pregnancy.[30]

The mother's blood pressure rises gradually as the pregnancy advances, increasing blood flow to the placenta and helping meet the baby's growing needs ... as long as uterine artery resistance is healthy. However, because monitoring the changing uterine artery over time is harder than keeping track of the umbilical artery, the first 10 years or so of Doppler research on the uterine artery were pretty much wasted. Uterine artery researchers frequently groped around just trying to find it with their equipment. They examined whatever blood vessel they found close to the placenta or under it. It was like working blind. When they went back after a week or so to examine the same vessel, they often couldn't see it where it was supposed to be because so much in the uterus had changed in the short time since the last examination. Also, while many researchers chose to study both the left and right uterine arteries, others chose to study only one of these, and some then specialized further by focusing on only one part of the artery before it starts splitting into thousands of ever-smaller vessels (many of which look maddeningly alike). Some researchers examined the left uterine artery in some patients and the right in others, depending on whichever artery was most accessible at the time. All this confusion created havoc when the research results were published. What were doctors to make of such a crazy-quilt of research results? They lacked enough consistency to bring them together logically and make sense of them. At the very least, it was all messy and inconvenient, and since doctors tend to hate mess and inconvenience and prefer things to be neat, organized and orderly, a controversy ensued as to whether, given all this confusion and disorder, it was worth the trouble to try to monitor the uterine artery with Doppler technology at all. This controversy is still alive today.

The Doppler research that's gone into this book encompasses consistent examinations of both uterine arteries of the patients because there are good indications that the left and right arteries have very different degrees of resistance to blood flow. This difference, my clinic's research has found, reflects the placenta's location. Some of our results have been published in a series of studies on how placental location affects pregnancy outcomes.[161-164]

Unfortunately, though, the general chaos surrounding Doppler studies of the uterine artery has led doctors to tend to ignore studies of this crucial placental vessel for years. Instead of trying to clarify the confusion surrounding Doppler studies of the uterine artery, obstetricians have simply backed away from the challenge of doing so, and in the process have effectively dismissed uterine artery Doppler monitoring as a test of fetal health. This is one of the worst scientific disasters of our age. For a doctor to ignore or dismiss information about the uterine artery is like ignoring or dismissing information about the fact that someone or something has interfered with a patient's ability to eat and breathe. Remember, uterine artery blood flow is a baby's primary source of food and oxygen. If this flow is impeded severely enough, the baby will die. If it's partly impeded, the baby's development will suffer in almost direct proportion. If the artery is around 50% impaired, the baby will grow about 50% less than it should.

Here's an example of how this can play out in real life. A 41-year-old woman became pregnant via in vitro fertilization (her egg was fertilized in a hospital laboratory and then implanted back inside her). After eight weeks, the hospital confirmed she had a viable pregnancy and released her to her obstetrician for routine care. That was Mistake Number One. For this patient and any such patient. To begin with, this pregnancy was very high-risk because of both the mother's age and the fact that it was a laboratory pregnancy. These factors immediately placed the mother at high risk of preterm birth, fetal growth retardation, fetal death and newborn death. High-risk specialists should have monitored this woman from Day One through the whole pregnancy. Yet she was managed like any other low-risk pregnancy. She had ultrasound testing at 12 weeks for Down syndrome and at 20 weeks for fetal anatomy. Both reports said the pregnancy was normal. When these reports were reviewed much later, not a single note about the placenta was in sight except that there was no placenta previa (where the placenta obstructs the cervix). There was no mention of placental quality or clots. But this wasn't because the placenta was normal. It was because it hadn't been examined. This is the standard of care today in America!

The patient was seen again four weeks after her 20-week ultrasound. This time the findings were grim. The baby's growth rate had dropped severely. Amniotic fluid was insufficient. Blood flow in the umbilical artery was impaired in a way which typically means impending death. The uterine artery showed severe blood flow reduction. These findings are consistent with complete failure of placental circulation. However, this degree of deterioration doesn't happen in four weeks unless there is a catastrophic placental abruption, which, in this case, hadn't happened. Extensive clinical evidence derived from other patient experiences indicates that the circumstances I've just described mean the abnormalities that were discovered at 24 weeks had most likely developed earlier and could probably have been detected at 20 weeks, if not before ... if only the placenta had been examined properly with ultrasound and Doppler. To make matters worse, this mother was examined by a high-risk specialist whose report said that although the uterine artery Doppler was abnormal at 24 weeks, "this finding is clinically insignificant." Well! Would it be clinically insignificant if someone kept their hand over your nose and mouth so you couldn't breathe or eat? This specialist ordered an amniocentesis and genetic tests to find out why the baby was small and suffering. But what about the placenta? And the baby's oxygen and food being cut off? At this stage there was still no mention of the placenta! No evaluation of placental size, appearance, evidence of damage or clotting. The specialist was just looking for exotic explanations. So what happened? I'd like to tell you it all worked out somehow. But it didn't. At 25 weeks the baby died. The patient was told "No more pregnancies" because her body was unfit to support a healthy pregnancy, even though the impressive (and expensive) genetic tests came back normal. I can't think of anything more demoralizing to tell a woman who is desperately trying to have a baby. And when it's factually wrong, I have no words to describe how outraged I feel. When this unlucky woman's placenta was eventually examined, it turned out to be severely growth-stunted, with evidence of clotting damage. In fact, it was a miracle the baby made it to 25 weeks.

The two biggest tragedies in this story are the following facts: First, signs that this kind of clotting damage is on the way can be seen as early as five weeks, if only the doctor looks for them. Second, such damage can be fixed with proper treatment, and the failure of the pregnancy can be prevented, if only the doctor takes these steps in good time. The enemy of this sort of pregnancy is the common myth that placental damage can't be repaired, a fable that not only harms babies but deceives mothers, leading them to feel that some inadequacy in themselves is somehow to blame when their baby dies or their pregnancy goes wrong in other ways. In fact, the word "myth" is too dignified a word for it. I use a stronger word for it: I call it a lie. And the destructiveness of the lie is made shockingly clear by this fact: this woman came to my clinic after the sad events I have described. My colleagues and I gave her the placental treatment that she needed … and she delivered a healthy eight-pound baby. So the story had a happy ending. However, what it says about the state of pregnancy healthcare in

America is deeply depressing.

So, given all the above information about misguided tests, what kind of testing can you rely on to protect your baby from placental failure? Many researchers in various scientific disciplines have helped us engage this question, often through studies of animals. As I've pointed out, animal research must be applied cautiously to human beings, but valuable information has come from the best of these studies. For example, studying seals has taught us about the "dive reflex." You've probably seen, at an aquarium or on TV, how seals take a deep breath before plunging, often staying underwater for a long time. They do this by changing their blood circulation to make maximum use of the oxygen from that one deep breath. They reduce blood supply to less essential organs while maintaining normal supply to their brain and to body areas responsible for rapid movement (to hunt fish or evade predators). Our understanding of this phenomenon in seals has given us insight into how human babies do something similar with brain-sparing. I've described in earlier pages how, when the baby's oxygen and food are severely reduced by a sudden catastrophe, brain-sparing kicks in. In an emergency it can compensate for oxygen deprivation for up to 10 minutes or so. If the mother is lucky enough to be in a hospital at the time, these minutes can be vital, giving doctors a chance to fix the emergency. But if the emergency strikes without help at hand, the baby usually dies. When placental failure isn't sudden but develops over days or weeks, brain-sparing can protect the baby from serious brain damage by constricting the vessels that deliver blood to organs including the liver, muscles, loose fatty tissues, bones, intestines and kidneys, and relaxing the blood vessels supplying oxygen and food to the brain, heart and adrenal glands. (Remember, the adrenals distribute hormones, the chemicals that tell much of the body what to do, and when.) Brain, heart and adrenals are key organs for the baby's immediate survival, and this kind of non-emergency brain-sparing can protect the baby for two to three weeks. It's amazing that this can happen at all, but make no mistake: it's not easy or good for the baby, whose blood pressure goes up. Its little heart has to work harder and harder. If it gets to the point where the heart itself doesn't get enough oxygen to cope with the extra work, the baby dies. So, one kind of testing that will definitely help you is monitoring blood vessel changes. If you get your doctor to do this, then, in the event of brain-sparing, action can be taken quickly to identify and, possibly, fix whatever triggered the brain-sparing. Your doctor must also assess the impact of the brain-sparing and decide whether the baby should be delivered prematurely. In the early stages of brain-sparing, the baby can compensate quite well. Its overall growth rate will likely slow down, but it can usually maintain normal growth for the brain, heart and adrenal glands. If the placenta declines beyond a certain point, however, the less essential organs will suffer increasingly and the baby may stop growing altogether, damaging its kidneys and intestines irreparably. Kidney failure may not be visible until the baby is born, because until then the placenta will do the kidneys' job. As far as the baby's intestine is concerned, if ongoing oxygen deprivation damages it severely, part of it may have to be removed shortly after birth. This surgery can be lethal. If brain-sparing kicks in after the 34th week, delivering the baby is best to prevent not only death but also severe development problems, including brain damage. If brain-sparing happens earlier than 34 weeks, it's more complicated, while under 32 weeks the risks associated with prematurity may damage the baby more than a limited amount of brain-sparing. In such cases, delaying delivery for even a few days might help the baby. In this situation, deciding exactly when to deliver is critical. All the baby's vital blood vessels must be monitored daily to determine when the heart will falter. That's when the baby must be delivered. If not, it will die. By the time the heart shows signs of failure, some brain damage has usually occurred, as well as severe damage to other vital organs.

In the late 1980s and early 1990s, doctors caring for patients with brain sparing, severe growth failure and severe placental damage under 32 weeks focused chiefly on the baby's survival rather than on its well-being in the event of survival. Patients were admitted to hospital for bed-rest, intense monitoring, and oxygen, with the principal aim of prolonging the pregnancy and giving the baby a chance to grow. This treatment seemed to make sense but it proved futile. Giving oxygen to the baby helped only temporarily, at the cost of misleading the doctors with a false impression of improvement. Worse, in many cases it actually harmed the baby: the oxygen infusion tricked the oxygen sensors in the baby's carotid arteries into registering that the crisis was over, causing brain-sparing to stop. This false all-clear signal instantly exposed the baby to brain damage. We now know that infusing oxygen into a placenta-compromised baby's blood is a devastating action. This realization in the 1990s defined my career. It was then that I finally understood that the only way to protect such babies was to prevent their predicaments from developing in the first place. In the years before I grappled with these brain-sparing challenges, I'd already seen placentas recover after being treated for clotting. Around the same time, tests became available to identify blood abnormalities responsible for placental damage. The certainty that clotting disorders caused such damage encouraged me to step up my use of blood-thinning treatments. To my great joy, the incidence of severe early growth retardation fell steadily and was eventually limited to patients who'd already reached this stage by the time they came to me. Where I was able to examine and treat a mother from early pregnancy, her baby's chances of developing severe growth retardation fell from 1 in 50 to less than 1 in 1000. Of my clinic's more than 15,000 at-risk patients at the time the research for this book was prepared, the number whose babies have developed early severe growth restriction was ...three! These results have attracted patients who have persistently suffered recurrent pregnancy loss despite treatments elsewhere, and recent years have seen a rise in the number of cases with severe immunity issues. This has led to the use of increasingly varied and more complex treatments. Since I deal almost entirely with high-risk patients, it's hard to know if this spike in complication diversity reflects a trend in the general population or simply means more of these patients are hearing about the good results and coming in so they and their babies can benefit from them. What I can say with confidence, however, is that these good results for patients are owed not to any special medical talent but entirely to the methods used, which I'm sure would work as well if they're properly applied in any clinic.

My team and I don't use the CST (contraction stress test, where the heart rate is measured while uterine contractions are induced, to determine how well the baby will cope with childbirth contractions) or NST (non-stress test, where the heart rate is monitored continuously without contraction inducement) at all, because we consider these tests to be ill-designed, with poor ability to assess a baby's health or forecast its risk of future suffering. For more than 20 years, all of our high-risk patients have been managed exclusively with a specially tailored mix of tests based on clinical experience and thousands of case studies.

This mix emphasizes early placental assessment, extensive use of Doppler and biophysical technology, and the earliest possible monitoring of placenta and fetus as they develop and adapt to the womb's changing environment. In the last few weeks, patients are examined weekly or more frequently if necessary, mapping the baby's condition with an array of blood-vessel studies. These ongoing evaluations of fetal and placental blood vessels help form a valuably integrated picture of the baby's health, risks and prospects. So, when you ask, "What kind of testing can I rely on to protect my baby to the fullest extent possible?" the answer is the combination of assessments I've just outlined. Your pregnancy's health, including your baby's present and future health and your own personal health during and after pregnancy, hardly ever hinges on a single thing. It's almost always part of a process that's complex in physiological space (i.e., in the number and distribution of physiological factors involved) as well as in time (i.e., most pregnancy factors don't come suddenly out of nowhere but develop over a long period, often going back to early events including the origins of the pregnancy or circumstances predating the pregnancy). By attending to this spatial and historical complexity, we can focus on the prevention of problems in a context of process. This is the guiding pregnancy management philosophy (the standard of care) that I recommend. The many successful, complicated-pregnancy outcomes in which I've been involved have owed their success, I believe, to this approach. Moreover, in the pregnancies I've studied where this approach hasn't been applied, I believe the lack of it has either caused the bad outcomes I've observed, or at least contributed to them significantly, or made things worse than they might have been. What all this boils down to is that there are today ways to avert pregnancy disaster and safely treat even patients who seem disaster-prone. By taking advantage of this knowledge, you can raise your chances of pregnancy success regardless of the pregnancy challenges you may be facing.

Chapter 25

MULTIPLE PREGNANCY

So far I've generally talked about "the baby" or "your baby" in the singular. This is because in natural pregnancies (without the help of fertility treatment) almost 99% of human mothers have one baby at a time. Although awareness of twins is wide in popular culture, they are rare, and more than two babies at once even rarer. However, in case a pregnancy lies in your future ,I want to tell you some things you need to know, starting with the fact that, in humans, multiple pregnancies are dangerous. Human bodies have evolved to have one baby at a time. In our species, multiple pregnancy happens only when they are caused by physiological abnormality, some fertility treatments, or other unusual circumstances, such as the occurrence of certain genes. Women normally produce one egg a month, but older mothers sometimes produce more, which raises the chances of multiple pregnancy. And if a woman receives two ore more embryos by means of Assisted Reproductive Technology (ART), her chances of having twins skyrocket, and could be as high as 20%.

In ART treatments, eggs are removed from the ovaries,

fertilized with sperm in a laboratory, then implanted back in the mother. Following the recent advent of pre-implantation genetic testing, ART clinics now transfer one embryo at a time. This reduces the chance of twins. There are two kinds of twins: identical (monozygotic) and non-identical (dizygotic or fraternal). In natural pregnancies, most twins (about 70%) are non-identical. If the twins have two separate placentas in two separate amniotic sacs, they can be either identical or non-identical. If they share a placenta, they can only be identical. Knowing what kind of twins they are is important because it affects their risk of birth defects and growth failure resulting from placental problems. Twins have almost twice the birth defect rate of natural single pregnancies, but many of these defects can be fixed. The biggest threats to identical twins sharing the same placenta are prematurity and growth failure due to a single placenta's inability to sustain two babies. Such twins and their mothers also face dangerous blood circulation problems.

Prematurity is a huge problem for twins. According to the World Health Organization report *Born Too Soon: The Global Action Report on Preterm Birth* (Geneva, 2012), multiple pregnancies have "nearly 10 times the risk of preterm birth compared to singleton births." (Because of the time taken to amass and then analyze public health statistics and finally get them into print, such numbers tend to be significantly out of date by the time they are published. For example, the WHO report I have just cited relies on figures originally published in 2006! I believe that since those statistics were assembled the situation has become worse.) Since we know that prematurity causes 80% of all newborn deaths and almost the same percentage of all long-term newborn illness, this means a large proportion of all twins are at risk of severe pregnancy complications, some of which are related to lifelong health problems. The past few decades have seen little progress in preventing prematurity. Many intensive care units for newborns have been improved, but premature babies still face grave problems. Evidence indicates twins delivered between 34 and 38 weeks do best.[165]

Although medical advances have significantly reduced the death rate of unborn and newborn babies, it remains high. In the 1970s about 10% of all twins died. It's now around 5%. But you have to read statistics carefully. Many studies of twin deaths ignore losses that happen under 32 weeks. This gives a misleadingly reassuring impression, and in my opinion is deeply offensive to the babies who die before 32 weeks. Don't they matter? Newborn twins also die and get sick more than single newborns. Some studies say the death and sickness rates for twins is up to 10% higher, but here again it's hard to know the real rate because most studies count only those babies who die within 30 days of birth, whereas intensive care units now often keep these babies alive beyond that point. Many of them die a little later, but because their deaths don't occur in the first 30 days, they're classified not as newborn deaths but as infant deaths. As a result, the United States has one of the highest infant mortality rates among developed countries.

Another problem is that because most women's bodies aren't equipped to nourish two babies simultaneously, placental abnormalities are more likely to cause growth failure in twins whether or not they're premature. Growth failure causes significant fetal and newborn death and illness. One of its forms is Twin-to-Twin Transfusion Syndrome (TTTS), where one twin develops acceptably but the other is stunted. Here we encounter another pregnancy myth. Many people have the idea that twins are "supposed" to be small, so why get upset? This is one of the most ridiculous concepts in obstetrics. There's no genetic or other physiological reason for twins to be associated with natural or intrinsic smallness relative to single babies. Growth restriction in a twin pregnancy shouldn't be passively accepted but should be regarded as an anomaly deserving treatment as aggressive as would be applied to any single fetus with growth restriction. Severe TTTS is very dangerous and often kills at least one of the twins. It can also kill both because, while one twin is stunted, the other can grow too much or too fast, with excessive amniotic fluid and body swelling. In severe cases of this kind, the probability of fetal death can be 70%. If the growth-rate difference between the twins exceeds 20%, early delivery should be prepared for and both fetuses should be monitored weekly, or more often, by Doppler and other means. But the longer delivery can be postponed, within desirable limits, the better. Unfortunately, the need for effective monitoring in such circumstances isn't helped by the methods currently used by most obstetricians, focused as these methods tend to be on saving the baby's life, with its health beyond survival coming second.

This focus on survival is partly because most severe cases of TTTS occur too early to allow the babies to be safely delivered. The key here is identifying the moment at which the risk to the babies in the womb exceeds the risk of premature delivery. But here's the crunch question: How is that moment determined? Currently, the popular policy (the standard of care) is to make this decision by using BPP (biophysical profile) and NST (electronic fetal non-stress test) monitoring. I've already talked about the weaknesses of these monitoring methods. Fetal well-being is usually taken to mean the baby is growing well, with enough food and oxygen. However,

MULTIPLE PREGNANCY

significant food insufficiency can be far less harmful than oxygen deprivation, which affects critical brain development. The NST evaluates heart activity in order to measure oxygen supply, but the heart is controlled from the brain, which is the main organ we must protect from oxygen starvation. So in concentrating on the heart, rather than on the brain, which controls the heart, the NST gathers information which is out of date by the time the doctor gets it. By the time the heart is affected, the brain has already been severely damaged. The use of the NST in this situation is thus bizarre and paradoxical. To make matters worse, about 95% of the time that the NST is classified as abnormal, it will likely be a false result, resulting in unnecessary medical intervention which may pose risks to both fetus and mother. So this is yet another reason why the NST should be eliminated from obstetric practice. Similar problems affect BPP testing, as we saw earlier.

The fetus's own carotid receptors (those tiny structures at the beginning of the carotid arteries, in the neck) are sensitive to the many problems that threaten the fetus in about 30% of all pregnancies. The receptors monitor the levels of oxygen, and send this information to the brain, which has the ability to respond by implementing brain-sparing if necessary. In keeping with the process-governed character of all fetal events, however, even a crisis response like brain-sparing isn't instant, like turning a switch. The brain is always receiving signals from the receptors and responding to them by sending orders to the blood vessels to adjust the supply of substances such as oxygen. This constant information exchange isn't just for crisis management but is part of the fetus's health management. It's like the action of the conductor of an orchestra, whose baton signals to various members of the orchestra to play their instruments louder or softer, slower or faster, depending on how the conductor assesses the overall weave of music that the whole orchestra is creating.

The baton represents a complex interplay between conductor and orchestra around which the entire musical process develops. In the fetus, this baton is the behavior of the blood: the speed of its flow in different parts of the fetal body at different times, its direction, its amount and the blood vessel resistance it meets. And we observe the baton by Doppler ultrasound. Regular Doppler monitoring, begun early enough, enables us to build a picture of the emerging pattern of the baby's development, detecting small, gradual but significant changes that may indicate oxygen supply problems long before it becomes necessary for the fetus to activate a major degree of brain-sparing. This can help identify the at-risk fetus before an oxygen supply problem reaches crisis proportions. Several studies in the 1990s helped my clinical colleagues and me to identify normal and abnormal patterns of blood flow redistribution in response to oxygen insufficiency. This work showed that fetal brain sparing doesn't happen in a single crisis mode but across a spectrum of health management responses over time; it is therefore these responses that must be monitored with Doppler from the earliest stages. At the first sign of any oxygen supply problems, the frequency of monitoring should be stepped up. The goal must be to enable us to time the delivery of the baby prematurely if this is unavoidable, yet still at an optimal moment within the context of prematurity, i.e. when brain-sparing is still in a moderate phase, to avoid brain injury. All this is necessary to determine as precisely as possible whether and, if applicable, when prematurity poses a bigger threat than some exposure to severe brain-sparing. Daily monitoring will then be necessary to decide an exact moment of optimal delivery.

I've been talking above mainly about the fate of the smaller, stunted identical twin in brain sparing cases, but the larger twin also has problems, you'll recall, although different ones: possible abnormal growth, excess blood, excess amniotic fluid, abnormal urine production, swelling, heart failure. The excess amniotic fluid compresses the umbilical veins and arteries, in turn reducing blood flow even further to both fetuses (who share a placenta, remember). The compression raises the baby's blood pressure, which in turn triggers various reflexes including a slowed and weakened heartbeat. The combination of blood circulation problems and body swelling (from water retention) affects the liver. If unchecked, this chain reaction of events can end in fetal death. The intricacy of fetal circulation tells us clearly, in my experience, that the only way to assess fetal health meaningfully is by early and regular Doppler examination of the circulatory system, which is currently the only test that really gives us usable advance insight into an approaching crisis. Doppler monitoring of the umbilical artery, umbilical vein, brain vessels, heart vessels, ductus venosus and descending aorta is very important in managing identical twins with Twin-to-Twin Transfusion Syndrome (TTTS) and non-identical twins with significant growth imbalance. (The risks are different in these two problems but the same information is needed to respond to them.) Umbilical artery Doppler is the most common fetal Doppler and is simple to do. It's excellent in predicting placenta weakness caused by blood vessel problems.

I've referred a lot to fetal heart failure. But what is heart failure? The "failing" heart typically goes on beating, but less and less strongly. This slows down the flow of blood, and the blood inside the heart exerts mounting pressure on the heart tissues as it waits to be pumped out. The effects of this include reducing oxygen and food provision to the brain and other organs, as well as a build-up of water in various parts of the body, which is called congestion, so the heart condition associated with it is commonly called congestive heart failure. This build-up of water isn't the same thing as a build-up of excess amniotic fluid in the sac of a bigger twin afflicted with TTTS. Amniotic fluid build-up is due solely to the bigger twin's receipt of excess blood at the expense of the stunted twin. Most TTTS cases are mild to moderate and respond well to amniocentesis, where some fluid is removed from the sac with a needle. A great deal of clinical experience indicates that some patients are cured with one amniocentesis; others need more. If amniocentesis fails to cure TTTS, three other possible steps can be considered: disrupting the membrane that separates the twin babies, thereby mixing the twins' amniotic fluid; using a laser beam to reduce the movement of blood from one twin to the other; or operating on the umbilical cord to control blood supply to one of the twins. Each of these methods has its own risks.

EPILOGUE

And that's how it is with pregnancy. There may always be a new problem around the corner, but new knowledge is becoming steadily available, even if doctors are slow to use it. With early enough monitoring, early enough treatment, and sufficient respect for the womb, especially the placenta, there's almost always a beacon of hope! Pregnancy contains extraordinary surprises and astonishing facts far exceeding the limits of conventional obstetric experience. In my opening pages, I noted that having a baby is one of the most complex experiences anyone can have, and I believe this has been borne out by everything I've shared with you. The complexity of the placenta, in particular, deserves a better deal from the medical profession. Neglect of this crucial organ has harmed the child-bearing interests of many women and their babies, and the babies they might have had. If you've turned to this book because you've already known heartache in these respects, or because you're struggling to have a child, know that you're not alone. Many women have shared your feelings and, despite my criticism of the medical establishment, there are many medical professionals who care deeply about your right to have a healthy baby. To express these feelings, and the principles and solidarity and determination they embody, you will find on Page 308 a statement that encapsulates much of what this book stands for. Please read it and share it with your friends.

This book doesn't really have an ending. At least, not in the way most books do. For practical reasons, I must come to the last page, but that won't bring an end to the things I've been discussing with you. If you're expecting a baby, or trying to get pregnant, or struggling to come to terms with a lost pregnancy, the fear of a loss, or just the question of what to do next, or if you're just looking ahead to a possible future pregnancy and seeking answers and groping with concerns or uncertainties, then this book is certainly not an ending. It's the beginning of a story yet to come, which you will write. This story will be your own adventure in the great and moving creation of new life. In embarking on your pregnancy journey, speak up about the fact that the latest placenta science offers us exciting, safe new ways to treat seemingly disaster-prone mothers and give them new hope. By doing so, you can not only put yourself on the path to overcoming any obstacles that stand between yourself and a successful pregnancy; you can also help women everywhere to do the same. Your body is rich in potential, no matter what anyone tells you to the contrary.

Take and retain full ownership of your pregnancy and of your parenting aspirations. If you talk enough to your friends and your doctor about what you've read here, you and other mothers can help stir so much discussion that no insurer or doctor will be able to ignore it indefinitely. Be motivated by the fact that pregnancy contains wonders beyond wonders, which can be challenging even for learned obstetricians who have grown used to dismissing whatever lies outside their comfort zones. Closed minds do ill service to mothers and babies, whose best interests can be served only if we approach the grand phenomenon of pregnancy with the awe and humility it deserves. As I hope this book has shown you, even in the apparently grimmest medical circumstances, the resources of a woman's body during pregnancy can achieve seeming miracles if we cooperate with them wisely.

Believe me, I have *seen* it happen.

THE PLACENTA BILL OF RIGHTS

Every woman's body contains the potential to grow a miraculous organ called the placenta. Unlike other organs, a placenta can't last a human lifetime. It is with you for a brief season. Then it is gone.

The placenta is the gateway between a mother and her unborn. In ways beyond counting, it nurtures the emerging life within, shaping its health not only in the womb but, to the extent of its power, for all years to come.

The placenta has no audible voice, yet in its own way it whispers to the new life, telling it what it must become. It holds the wisdom of creation. When a newborn cries its greeting to the world, those who glance upon the placenta's discarded, soon-forgotten substance may not realize they are glimpsing the fingerprints of God.

Like all living things, the placenta is not an island, sufficient in itself. It needs sustenance and the support of such knowledge as our kind has managed to amass. Therefore, let it be known that the placenta, too, has rights, which the mother must claim for it in her pregnancy's name:

1.
The right to be acknowledged as the lifeline between mother and unborn child, and as the key to the pregnancy's success.

2.
The right to be examined from the outset of the pregnancy, by all the best means available to physicians, so as to help achieve a full-term pregnancy culminating in the birth of a child healthy enough to realize its full genetic potential; and such monitoring must continue frequently and regularly throughout the pregnancy to ensure that placenta health is optimally sustained, regardless of whether such examination and sustenance is in the financial interest of any commercial entity.

3.
The right to be recognized as a treatable organ whose disorders are subject to correction and prevention, and to receive such treatment as needed from the earliest phases of the pregnancy, in good time and with all medicinal and technological resources, with the full benefit of such diagnostic and remedial treatment as may be needed to identify in good time, eliminate, and prevent, all placental illness.

4.
The right to be extensively examined after birth, so that, through such examination, medical practitioners shall obtain such information about the placenta and the pregnancy as may be relevant to the continuing health of the mother, the baby and any pregnancy to follow.

5.
The right to be the full and thorough subject of medical instruction, training and continuing education for all medical practitioners concerned with pregnancy care, so that such they shall be properly equipped to provide the most informed pregnancy care possible, in the light of research findings and knowledge derived from clinical experience.

6.
The right to be the subject of the highest research and knowledge development priorities, and of such changes in practice and standard of care as are necessary to reflect technological innovation and the growth of clinical knowledge, regardless of whether such changes are convenient to health care industry managers.

7.
The right to a thoughtful and enduring acknowledgement, not only theoretical but carried through and applied in diagnosis, preventive care and treatment, that the placenta, like the fetus, is the product of both paternal and maternal genes.

To these precepts, all responsible medical practitioners and providers of medical services, including hospitals, insurers, lawmakers and all health care institutions and enterprises, private and public, are bound, in conscience, in conduct, and in dedication to the health of mothers, fetuses and newborns everywhere.

It's *your* pregnancy. In *your* body. Believe in it.

Index

A

abdominal pressure 134
abortion 77, 91, 220
accessory lobe 135
ACE insertion/deletion gene mutation 220
ACOG (the American College of Obstetricians and Gynecologists) 248
adrenal glands 25, 267, 291, 292
African-American 174
afterbirth 6, 27
AIDS (acquired immunodeficiency syndrome) 125
albumin 116
allantois 72, 73
alpha2-antiplasmin 222
Alzheimer's 203
American Heart Association 255
amino acids 115, 272
amniocentesis 134, 135, 140, 141
amniotic fluid 113, 128, 142, 148, 240, 243, 256, 264, 282, 283, 284, 300, 303, 304
Amniotic fluid 289
anemic, anemia 16, 118, 149
anesthesia 24, 228, 229
anesthesiologist 229, 230
Annexin V 221
anti-annexin V antibodies 221
antibodies 56, 61, 120, 121, 168, 212, 213, 221, 222
anti-clotting medication 27, 184, 186, 187, 197, 223, 227, 228, 254, 255
anticoagulant 21, 102, 225, 228, 243
anti-contraction 104
anticonvulsant 123, 124
antidepressant 125, 270
anti-inflammatory 104, 134
antioxidant 95
antithrombin III 209, 211, 221
antiviral 125, 126
anxiety 3, 26, 228, 270, 271

aorta 65, 66, 240, 303
APS (antiphospholipd antibody syndrome) 168
arcuate arteries 66
ARDS (Adult Respiratory Distress Syndrome) 268
Aristotle 76
arrhythmia 123, 283
aspirin 101, 132, 134, 144, 187, 190, 193, 197, 221, 227, 228, 243, 285
Athens, Greece 35
atony 151
atrium 17, 64, 65
autism 271
auto-immune disorder 56, 121, 192, 193

B

bad eggs 189
Barker, David 32, 33, 34, 35, 36, 37
Barker Hypothesis (fetal programming hypothesis) 32
basilar arteries 67
bed rest 102, 148, 243
beta-blocker 123
beta-HCG (beta chain of chorionic gonadotropin) 178
bicuspid valve 65
bifurcated (bicornuate) uterus 21
birth canal 132, 133
birth defects 298
blastocyst 68, 102
bleeding 22, 23, 97, 99, 100, 101, 102, 124, 133, 134, 135, 136, 145, 148, 149, 150, 151, 155, 158, 161, 162, 175, 193, 208, 220, 226, 227, 228, 243
bleeding, sporadic 99, 145
blindness 46, 106, 245
blocked tubes 189
blocking antibodies 56
blood bank 151
blood loss 149, 150, 162
blood pressure 83, 88, 114, 148, 149, 153, 162, 194, 243, 274, 285, 286, 292, 303
blood sugar 211, 283
blood thinner 101
blood transfusion 16, 150, 161
BMJ (Journal of the British Medical Association) 32

BPP (biophysical profile) 240, 282, 283, 284, 300, 301
brain 16, 17, 20, 25, 26, 27, 28, 29, 81, 88, 113, 117, 118, 120, 123, 124, 127, 136, 142, 143, 147, 149, 176, 203, 204, 227, 240, 256, 264, 265, 266, 267, 268, 269, 271, 274, 275, 278, 279, 284, 291, 292, 293, 300, 301, 302, 303
brain damage 20, 88, 142, 149, 227, 256, 266, 267, 268, 269, 274, 275, 284, 291, 292, 293
brain-sparing 291, 292, 293, 301, 302
Braxton-Hicks contractions 273
breast-fed 121

C

cancer 32, 117, 173, 202, 203, 206, 227
 cancer, breast 202, 206
cancer-causing substances 117
Canick, Jack 140
capillaries 129, 285
carbon dioxide 58, 61, 112, 267, 283
cardiovascular disease 35, 85, 122, 203, 204, 205, 206, 207, 208
 studies focusing primarily on men 205
 women's risk of death 206
carotid arteries 293, 301
carotid receptors 301
catheter 145, 150
Caucasian 174
Centers for Disease Control and Prevention 252
cerebral palsy 88, 99, 106, 113, 154, 156, 226, 245, 252, 254, 264, 265, 270, 279, 281, 284
cerebrospinal fluid 127
cervical cerclage 104, 226
cervical shortening 104, 221
cervix 58, 104, 105, 133, 134, 135, 143, 161, 168, 170, 184, 226, 241, 242, 243, 244, 246, 256, 289
cesarean section 20, 227, 243, 278
cholesterol 203, 204
chorioamnionitis 256
chorion 24, 190
chorionic villi 24, 190, 221, 225, 226
chromosomal defects 164
chromosome 164, 168, 173, 176
cilia 53

cinderella embryo 55
Clay, D 146
clot 27, 28, 29, 59, 60, 97, 113, 136, 150, 155, 175, 193, 210, 223, 256
cocaine 148, 268
Cochrane Collaboration Group 279
collagen 256
conception 2, 21, 43, 52, 68, 74, 78, 83, 144, 260, 267, 272
congestive heart failure 304
constipation 134
copper 118
costs, administrative 260
costs, hospital 155
Couvelaire, Alexandre 150
couvelaire uterus 150
creatinine 149
cross-membrane transfer 115
CST (contraction stress test) 278, 279, 294
Curie, Marie 89
CVS (chorionic villus sampling) 140, 145, 146
  transabdominal 146
  transcervical 145

D

D'amico, K 146
Darwin, Charles 89, 90
dead cells 256
death
  newborn 181, 284, 288, 299
death of the mother 154
death rate 85, 167, 207, 239, 299
decidua 256
deformity 124
depression 167, 268, 271
developmental delays 106, 113
diabetes 32, 117, 165, 166, 190, 204, 205, 211, 220, 223, 252, 267, 283
diagnosis 27, 84, 96, 97, 99, 136, 140, 144, 151, 164, 250, 254, 307
diastolic 103, 109
diet 117, 205, 269, 271
diffusion 128
digitalis 123
digoxin 123

disabled 156
dive reflex 291
doppler 16, 17, 132, 135, 149, 153, 184, 185, 186, 197, 198, 221, 225,
    236, 238, 240, 248, 250, 251, 274, 275, 278, 284, 285, 286, 287,
    288, 289, 295, 300, 302, 303
  CDI (color doppler imaging) 285
  CWD (continuous-wave doppler) 285
  Doppler, Christian 132
  PWD (pulsed-wave doppler) 285
double standard 183
down syndrome 140, 141, 164, 173, 176, 178, 278, 288
drugs 119, 120, 122, 123, 124, 125, 126, 226, 227, 228
ducks 121
ductus venosus 16, 17, 303
DVT (deep vein thrombosis) 223

E

early pregnancy loss 99
eclampsia 88, 99, 113, 148, 153, 154, 155, 156, 169, 176, 177, 221, 222,
    226, 239, 252, 253, 254, 256, 261, 270, 273, 275
Edward's syndrome (trisomy 18) 164
egg 52, 194, 288, 297
embryo 53, 54, 55, 56, 57, 58, 59, 66, 67, 68, 69, 71, 72, 73, 74, 81, 82, 93,
    94, 95, 97, 102, 131, 164, 169, 220, 222, 272
  implantation 220
emotion 68
endocytosis 112
endometrium 52, 53, 54, 55, 56, 66, 67, 69, 74, 86, 93
enoxaparin sodium 101, 144, 243
Environmental Working Group 272
epidemiologist 34, 37
epidural 24, 228, 229
  anesthesia, safety, availability and denial of 228, 229
epigenetic imprinting 94, 95
epilepsy 123
estrogen 129
ethnicity 174
evidence
  clinical 168, 225
  scientific 28
excessive clotting 155, 209, 221, 227

exocytosis 113

F

facial expressions 125
Factor II 211
Factor VIII 208
Factor V Leiden 211
fallopian tube 52, 53
Falloppio, Gabriele 53
false positives 140
false reading 103, 109
Fantastic Voyage 59
father 21, 48, 52, 56, 132, 157, 215, 216, 243, 247
fatty acid 116, 117
fear 23, 40, 129, 171, 228, 229
feminism 206
fetal
  asphyxia 23, 142, 270
  blood 52
  bowel 284
  breathing 283
  cardiology 104
  circulation 26, 303
  circumference 118
  death / demise 17, 28, 99, 133, 142, 169, 176, 181, 222, 226, 239, 264, 278, 279, 284, 288, 300, 303
  hydrocephalus 143, 145
  hypoxia 113, 124, 283, 284
  nuchal area 140
  waste 112
fetoscope 278
fibrinogen 222
fibroids 171
fish 117, 291
fish oil 117
folic acid 193
foods
  processed 117, 271, 272
  whole 117, 272
forceps 278
Fran's story 189

FTV (fetal thrombotic vasculopathy) 177

G

gender bias 205
genes 33, 56, 85, 87, 94, 127, 129, 164, 169, 175, 176, 205, 216, 297, 307
genetic mutation 144, 173
genetic potential 37, 87, 94, 306
genital tract 168
gestational age 259
gestational sac 73
gland 112, 129
glomerulonephritis 148
glucose 60, 114, 115
God's will explanation of miscarriage 84
Graduation Theory 79
Greene, Michael 281
gums 149
gynecologist 27, 101, 193

H

handicaps 144, 145, 205, 262
HCG (human chorionic gonadotropin) 129, 195, 196
health care policy 203, 253
heart 3, 16, 17, 22, 25, 26, 32, 44, 60, 62, 63, 64, 65, 88, 103, 104, 107, 108, 114, 120, 122, 123, 125, 136, 150, 153, 165, 166, 176, 184, 185, 186, 203, 204, 207, 232, 240, 245, 259, 265, 267, 278, 279, 281, 282, 283, 291, 292, 293, 294, 301, 303, 304
heartbeat 23, 278, 303
heart disease 32, 122, 123
heart failure 122, 303, 304
heavy lifting 134
helicine arteries 67
hematologist 210
hemoglobin 149
hemophilia 208
hemorrhage 158
heparin 187, 197, 221, 225, 227, 228, 230
hepatitis 121
high blood pressure 83, 88, 148
high-risk pregnancy 2, 10, 15, 39, 49, 105, 111, 141, 192, 207, 260
hiv (human immunodeficiency virus) 125, 126

home pregnancy test kit 194
Hon, Edward H 278
hormones 25, 60, 129, 205, 277, 291
hot spot 54
hunger 129, 233
hydramnios 148
hydrocephalus 143, 145
hydrops 16
hypertension 32, 117, 122, 123, 148, 149, 166, 204, 205, 211, 221, 223, 264, 267
hypofibrinolysis 220
hysterectomy 134, 150
hysterotomy 134

I

ibuprofen 134
iliac arteries 66
immune system 25, 27, 56, 61, 96, 97, 98, 102, 121, 148, 168, 169, 174, 190, 191, 192, 196, 212, 223, 225, 256
immunoglobulins 120
indomethacin 104, 122, 243, 245
infant mortality 250, 299
infection 121, 122, 148, 154, 168, 242, 243, 256
inferior vena cava 17
infertility 83, 117, 139, 171, 222
inflammation 143, 154, 168, 225, 246
insulin 165, 220
insurance 7, 8, 9, 10, 12, 152, 167, 182, 185, 202, 205, 219, 231, 235, 245, 246, 247, 248, 249, 250, 251, 257, 262
intelligence 205, 271
intercourse 134
intervillous space 52, 58, 67, 72, 74, 75, 95, 96, 98, 112, 179, 212, 221, 225, 238, 269
intestine 292
IUGR (intrauterine growth restriction) 87, 254
ischemia 104, 154, 256
IUI (intrauterine insemination) 139, 144
IVG (in vitro fertilization) 83, 189, 190, 193, 194

J

Jehovah's Witness 161

INDEX

journals 111, 187, 255, 261

K

kidneys 26, 66, 208, 243, 291, 292
King, K 146
Kofinas Perinatal 37
Kofinas website 272

L

labor 22, 23, 49, 104, 122, 126, 133, 134, 135, 139, 148, 154, 155, 156, 158, 170, 183, 184, 193, 196, 226, 228, 229, 242, 244, 257, 270, 273, 274, 278, 279
  premature 104, 122, 196, 226
laser 59, 304
late fetal death 99
lawsuits 225
lesions 239, 240
liability 228
lifeline 30, 306
lipid 25, 102, 106, 107, 108, 109, 191, 193
lipoprotein 116, 222
Little, William 264
LMWH (low molecular weigh herapin) 197, 221, 223, 225, 226, 228, 229, 230, 237, 254
lungs 22, 64, 88, 109, 113, 114, 134, 149, 210, 223, 245, 267, 268
lupus 148

M

magnesium sulfate 183, 226
manganese 117
Mary's story 29
maternal anatomical problems 170
maternal clotting 27
maternal-fetal specialist (perinatologist) 205, 211, 234
Mediterranean diet 117
menstrual period 57
metabolism 58
midwife 278
Miranda's choice 101
miscarriage 2, 8, 38, 43, 44, 46, 68, 74, 134, 141, 154, 156, 162, 163, 164,

319

165, 166, 167, 168, 169, 170, 171, 173, 174, 175, 176, 216, 217, 226, 231
misinformation 4, 9, 38
mitral valve 65
molar pregnancy 173
molybdenum 117
morula 68
MS-AFP (maternal serum alpha-fetoprotein) 176, 177, 178, 181
MTHFR (4g/5g (pai-1) gene mutation 220
multiple pregnancy 297
muscle cells 57, 71
muscle relaxants 122
muscles 26, 63, 124, 158, 266, 291
myomectomy 171
myometrium 66, 67

N

National Institutes of Health 252
NK cells 25, 169, 237
neonatal death 83
nerves 63, 123, 124, 268
nervous system 16, 57, 94, 117, 123, 124, 125, 129, 135
neurological 81, 123, 265, 269, 270, 279
neurologist 124
neurotransmitter 125, 268, 270
New England Journal of Medicine 279, 281
nifedipine 104, 122, 194, 243
non-steroidal anti-inflammatory 134, 243
non-stress test 186, 240, 278, 294
nuchal translucency 139
nucleus 52
nutrients 24, 26, 31, 51, 52, 54, 60, 66, 72, 96, 97, 112, 113, 130, 273

O

Oakley, Ann 44
obesity 32, 117, 175
OBGYN (obstetrician-gynecologist) 101, 146
obstetrician 152
obstetrician's Irony 152
OECD (organization for economicCo-operation and development) 165, 249

olive oil 117
omega-6 117
open-heart surgery 165
ovarian cysts 220
ovaries 53, 129, 298
ovulation 53, 54, 194, 195
oxygenation 26, 275
oxygen deprivation 28, 87, 113, 124, 149, 154, 266, 274, 291, 292, 300

P

pain 136, 228, 242, 243
  abdominal 136
PAPP-A (pregnancy associated plasma protein a) 140, 145, 178, 179, 180, 181, 182, 183, 184, 186, 187, 197, 198
pathologist 192
phospholipids 168, 212
placenta
  low-lying 133, 161
  off-center (unilateral) 274
placenta abruption 135
Placenta Bill of Rights 305
placenta blind spot 6, 86
placental barrier membrane 113, 114
placental bed 152
placental damage 27, 113, 132, 157, 177, 180, 181, 193, 212, 225, 226, 239, 243, 244, 266, 290, 293
placental lake 177
placental syndrome 259, 260
placenta previa 100, 132, 133, 134, 136, 289
placenta separation 99
plaque 203, 204
plasma 60, 61, 116, 128, 140, 178
platelets 60, 222, 227, 228
poison 118
pollution 117
prednisone 102, 103
preeclampsia 83, 153, 181, 239, 253, 254, 255, 264
pregnancy failure rate 1, 10, 19
pregnancy hormone 195
pregnancy opportunity window 217
prejudice against motherhood 231

preterm birth 99, 113, 154, 155, 156, 168, 169, 176, 181, 221, 226, 253, 254, 256, 288, 298
profit 9, 167, 262, 272
progesterone 101, 129, 273
programming 32
protein 60, 114, 115, 116, 120, 140, 149, 178, 208, 209, 211, 221, 222
protein C 209, 211, 221
protein S 208, 209, 211, 221
protein Z 222
pulmonary embolism 210, 223

R

radial arteries 66, 67
red cells 60, 61, 62, 73, 114, 284
reproductive endocrinologist 189
reproductive immunologist 102
research 33, 34, 36, 89, 90, 111, 153, 177, 202, 205, 206, 232, 255, 274, 279, 280, 286, 287, 291, 294, 307
respiratory sinus arrhythmia 283
Roe versus Wade 77
Ruth's Story 241

S

saliva 277
schizophrenia 271
scleroderma 148
seafood 117, 271
seals 291
seizure 124
selenium 118
selfhood 39
septum 170
serotonin 125, 268, 269, 270, 271
sexual stimulation 129
Shelley's story 139
shock 23, 151
silver bullet 253
singleton 255, 298
skull 127
smoking 90
sonogram 23, 243

sound waves 136, 284
Spencer, Herbert 89, 90
sperm 52, 298
spina bifida 176, 178
spiral arteries 55, 57, 58, 59, 67, 71, 72, 74, 82, 95, 97, 148, 152, 158, 220, 272, 273
spiral artery plugs 74
spiral artery remodeling 87, 99, 112, 220, 236
spotting (sporadic bleeding) 99, 145
SSRI (selective serotonin reuptake inhibitors) 125
standard of care 104, 183, 184, 186, 187, 211, 212, 213, 249, 280, 289, 295, 300, 307
steroid (corticosteroid) 22, 102, 193, 197
stethoscope 278
stillborn 99
stomach 208, 252, 266
stress 49, 98, 104, 106, 123, 125, 140, 143, 182, 186, 202, 204, 216, 240, 278, 294, 300
stroke 122, 142, 147, 204
sugar 114, 211, 283
survival of the fittest 88, 89, 90
swelling 16, 300, 303
symbiosis 153
syncytium 112

T

TAT (thrombin-antithrombin complex) 155
terbutaline 183, 226
thalidomide 119
thrifty gene 175
thrombin 155
thrombophilia 21, 22, 24, 28, 101, 102, 132, 144, 145, 147, 148, 149, 155, 184, 187, 190, 191, 196, 208, 209, 210, 212, 215, 216, 217, 218, 220, 240, 243, 247
thrombosis 96, 99, 131, 132, 142, 147, 149, 177, 178, 186, 221, 223, 225, 226
thyroid 118, 166
Time Magazine 32
T, McGuiness 146
tocolytic 104
trace elements 118

transporter molecule 116
trimester
  first 73, 88, 91, 99, 154, 220, 264
  second 171
trimester myth 88, 90
trimester zero 78
triplets 255
Trisomy 18 (Edward's Syndrome) 164
tryptophan 269, 270, 271, 272
TTTS (twin-to-twin transfusion syndrome) 299, 300, 303, 304
twins
  identical (monozygotic) 298, 303
  non-identical (dizgotic or fraternal) 303

U

ultrasound 5, 21, 23, 73, 86, 96, 99, 104, 108, 109, 111, 113, 131, 132, 134, 135, 136, 139, 142, 144, 145, 149, 150, 153, 158, 177, 178, 179, 184, 186, 190, 197, 198, 221, 238, 242, 243, 263, 282, 284, 286, 288, 289, 302
  transvaginal 184
umbilical artery 20, 28, 103, 109, 131, 237, 238, 248, 284, 285, 286, 289, 303
umbilical cord
  eccentric 131
  short 148
umbilical vein 16, 20, 130, 238, 303
umbilicus 75
urine 128, 149, 277, 303
uterine artery 23, 59, 66, 67, 255, 273, 284, 286, 287, 288, 289
uterine cavity 53, 97

V

vacuum extraction 278
vaginal birth 133, 143
valproate 124
vasa previa 132, 133, 135
vegetables 95, 117, 271, 272
ventricle 16, 64, 65
vibroacoustic stimulator 280, 281
vitamin B 144

W

waste products 58
water 60, 65, 71, 113, 115, 127, 128, 197, 242, 303, 304
white blood cells 73, 120, 225, 256

Y

yolk sac 72, 73, 112

Z

zinc 118
zygote 68

REFERENCES

1. Bick, R.L., *Recurrent miscarriage syndrome and infertility caused by blood coagulation protein or platelet defects*. Hematol Oncol Clin North Am, 2000. **14**(5): p. 1117-31.
2. Kofinas, A., M. Cabbad, and G. Kofinas, *Ductus venosus flow velocity in acute fetal congestive heart failure during fetal transfusion*. J Matern Fetal Invest, 1996(6): p. 188-189.
3. Cheema, R., M. Dubiel, and S. Gudmundsson, *Fetal brain sparing is strongly related to the degree of increased placental vascular impedance*. J Perinat Med, 2006. **34**(4): p. 318-22.
4. Roza, S.J., et al., *What is spared by fetal brain-sparing? Fetal circulatory redistribution and behavioral problems in the general population*. Am J Epidemiol, 2008. **168**(10): p. 1145-52.
5. Barker, D.J. and C. Osmond, *Infant mortality, childhood nutrition, and ischaemic heart disease in England and Wales*. Lancet, 1986. **1**(8489): p. 1077-81.
6. Barker, D.J., et al., *The relation of small head circumference and thinness at birth to death from cardiovascular disease in adult life*. BMJ, 1993. **306**(6875): p. 422-6.
7. Barker, D.J., et al., *Weight in infancy and death from ischaemic heart disease*. Lancet, 1989. **2**(8663): p. 577-80.
8. De Boo, H. and J. Harding, *The developmental origins of adult disease (Barker) hypothesis*. Aust N Z J Obstet Gynaecol, 2006. **46**: p. 4-14.
9. Arriaza B., A.M., and Gerszten E., *Maternal Mortality in Pre-Columbian Indians of Arica, Chile*. American Journal of Physical Anthropology, 1988. **77**: p. 6.
10. (OECD), O.f.E.C.a.D., *Mean age of women at first childbirth*. http://www.oecd.org/els/soc/SF_2_3_Age_mothers_childbirth.pdf, 2017.
11. Martin, C.B., Jr. and E.M. Ramsey, *Gross anatomy of the placenta of rhesus monkeys*. Obstet Gynecol, 1970. **36**(2): p. 167-77.
12. Ramsey, E.M. and M.W. Donner, *Placenta Vascular and Circulation: anatomy, physiology, radiology, clinical aspects*. Atlas and Textbook. 1980, Philadelphia-London-Toronto: W.B. Saunders Company, Georg Thieme Publishers Stutgart.
13. Minas, V., D. Loutradis, and A. Makrigiannakis, *Factors controlling blastocyst implantation*. Reprod Biomed Online, 2005. **10**(2): p. 205-16.
14. Murphy, C.R., *Understanding the apical surface markers of uterine receptivity: pinopods-or uterodomes?* Hum Reprod, 2000. **15**(12): p. 2451-4.
15. Nardo, L.G., T.C. Li, and R.G. Edwards, *Introduction: human embryo implantation failure and recurrent miscarriage: basic science and clinical practice*. Reprod Biomed Online, 2006. **13**(1): p. 11-2.
16. Paria, B.C., et al., *Molecular signaling in uterine receptivity for implantation*.

Semin Cell Dev Biol, 2000. **11**(2): p. 67-76.

17. Laird, S.M., E.M. Tuckerman, and T.C. Li, *Cytokine expression in the endometrium of women with implantation failure and recurrent miscarriage.* Reprod Biomed Online, 2006. **13**(1): p. 13-23.

18. Tranguch, S., et al., *Molecular complexity in establishing uterine receptivity and implantation.* Cell Mol Life Sci, 2005. **62**(17): p. 1964-73.

19. Quenby, S. and R. Farquharson, *Uterine natural killer cells, implantation failure and recurrent miscarriage.* Reprod Biomed Online, 2006. **13**(1): p. 24-8.

20. Ledee-Bataille, N., *[Materno-foetal dialogue and human embryo implantation: some evolving concepts].* J Gynecol Obstet Biol Reprod (Paris), 2004. **33**(7): p. 564-76.

21. Hoozemans, D.A., et al., *Human embryo implantation: current knowledge and clinical implications in assisted reproductive technology.* Reprod Biomed Online, 2004. **9**(6): p. 692-715.

22. Fazleabas, A.T., J.J. Kim, and Z. Strakova, *Implantation: embryonic signals and the modulation of the uterine environment—a review.* Placenta, 2004. **25 Suppl A**: p. S26-31.

23. Whitley, G.S. and J.E. Cartwright, *Trophoblast-mediated spiral artery remodelling: a role for apoptosis.* J Anat, 2009. **215**(1): p. 21-6.

24. Pijnenborg, R., L. Vercruysse, and M. Hanssens, *The uterine spiral arteries in human pregnancy: facts and controversies.* Placenta, 2006. **27**(9-10): p. 939-58.

25. Ashton, S.V., et al., *Uterine spiral artery remodeling involves endothelial apoptosis induced by extravillous trophoblasts through Fas/FasL interactions.* Arterioscler Thromb Vasc Biol, 2005. **25**(1): p. 102-8.

26. Teasdale, F., *Gestational changes in the functional structure of the human placenta in relation to fetal growth: a morphometric study.* Am J Obstet Gynecol, 1980. **137**(5): p. 560-8.

27. Hafner, E., et al., *Placental growth from the first to the second trimester of pregnancy in SGA-foetuses and pre-eclamptic pregnancies compared to normal foetuses.* Placenta, 2003. **24**(4): p. 336-42.

28. Proctor, L.K., et al., *Placental size and the prediction of severe early-onset intrauterine growth restriction in women with low pregnancy-associated plasma protein-A.* Ultrasound Obstet Gynecol, 2009. **34**(3): p. 274-82.

29. Smith, G.C., et al., *First-trimester placentation and the risk of antepartum stillbirth.* JAMA, 2004. **292**(18): p. 2249-54.

30. Kofinas, A.D., et al., *Uteroplacental Doppler flow velocity waveform indices in normal pregnancy: a statistical exercise and the development of appropriate reference values.* Am

REFERENCES

J Perinatol, 1992. **9**(2): p. 94-101.

31. Ray, J.G., et al., *Cardiovascular health after maternal placental syndromes (CHAMPS): population-based retrospective cohort study.* Lancet, 2005. **366**(9499): p. 1797-803.

32. Quenby, S., et al., *Recurrent miscarriage and long-term thrombosis risk: a case-control study.* Hum Reprod, 2005. **20**(6): p. 1729-32.

33. Wintermark, P., et al., *Fetal placental thrombosis and neonatal implications.* Am J Perinatol, 2010. **27**(3): p. 251-6.

34. Sebire, G., *Factor V Leiden as a cause of hemiplegic cerebral palsy, neonatal stroke, and placental thrombosis?* Ann Neurol, 1998. **44**(3): p. 426-7.

35. Kraus, F.T. and V.I. Acheen, *Fetal thrombotic vasculopathy in the placenta: cerebral thrombi and infarcts, coagulopathies, and cerebral palsy.* Hum Pathol, 1999. **30**(7): p. 759-69.

36. Bendon, R.W., S. Bornstein, and O.M. Faye-Petersen, *Two fetal deaths associated with maternal sepsis and with thrombosis of the intervillous space of the placenta.* Placenta, 1998. **19**(5-6): p. 385-9.

37. Kraus, F.T., *Placenta: thrombosis of fetal stem vessels with fetal thrombotic vasculopathy and chronic villitis.* Pediatr Pathol Lab Med, 1996. **16**(1): p. 143-8.

38. Rolschau, J., *Infarctions and Intervillous Thrombosis in Placenta, and Their Association with Intrauterine Growth Retardation.* Acta Obstet Gynecol Scand, 1978. **57**(S72): p. 22-27.

39. Fox, H., *Thrombosis of foetal arteries in the human placenta.* J Obstet Gynaecol Br Commonw, 1966. **73**(6): p. 961-5.

40. Jauniaux, E., et al., *Trophoblastic oxidative stress in relation to temporal and regional differences in maternal placental blood flow in normal and abnormal early pregnancies.* Am J Pathol, 2003. **162**(1): p. 115-25.

41. Kofinas, A., G. Kofinas, and V. Sutija, *The role of second trimester ultrasound in the diagnosis of placental hypoechoic lesions leading to poor pregnancy outcome.* J Matern Fetal Neonatal Med, 2007. **20**(12): p. 859-66.

42. Barclay, D., K. Evans, and R. Fox, *Ultrasound-diagnosed placental infarction in a woman with recurrent fetal growth restriction.* J Obstet Gynaecol, 2005. **25**(2): p. 200-1.

43. Zaidi, S.F., et al., *Comprehensive Imaging Review of Abnormalities of the Placenta.* Ultrasound Q, 2016. **32**(1): p. 25-42.

44. Abramowicz, J.S. and E. Sheiner, *Ultrasound of the placenta: a systematic approach, Part I: Imaging.* Placenta, 2008. **29**(3): p. 225-40.

45. Jaffe, R. and J.R. Woods, Jr., *Color Doppler imaging and in vivo assessment of*

the anatomy and physiology of the early uteroplacental circulation. Fertil Steril, 1993. **60**(2): p. 293-7.

46. Kofinas, A. and J. Kofinas, *Indomethacin as a diagnostic and therapeutic tool in the management of progressive cervical shortening diagnosed by trans-vaginal sonography.* J Matern Fetal Neonatal Med, 2010.

47. Evans, D.J., A.D. Kofinas, and K. King, *Intraoperative amniocentesis and indomethacin treatment in the management of an immature pregnancy with completely dilated cervix.* Obstet Gynecol, 1992. **79**(5 (Pt 2)): p. 881-2.

48. Pacifici, G.M., *Placental transfer of antibiotics administered to the mother: a review.* Int J Clin Pharmacol Ther, 2006. **44**(2): p. 57-63.

49. Pacifici, G.M., *Transfer of antivirals across the human placenta.* Early Hum Dev, 2005. **81**(8): p. 647-54.

50. Muller-Schmehl, K., et al., *Localization of alpha-tocopherol transfer protein in trophoblast, fetal capillaries' endothelium and amnion epithelium of human term placenta.* Free Radic Res, 2004. **38**(4): p. 413-20.

51. Holcberg, G., et al., *New aspects in placental drug transfer.* Isr Med Assoc J, 2003. **5**(12): p. 873-6.

52. Heikkinen, T., U. Ekblad, and K. Laine, *Transplacental transfer of amitriptyline and nortriptyline in isolated perfused human placenta.* Psychopharmacology (Berl), 2001. **153**(4): p. 450-4.

53. Schneider, H. and M. Proegler, *Placental transfer of beta-adrenergic antagonists studied in an in vitro perfusion system of human placental tissue.* Am J Obstet Gynecol, 1988. **159**(1): p. 42-7.

54. Chamberlain, G. and A. Wilkinson, *Placental Transfer.* 1979.

55. Bissonnette, J.M., et al., *Glucose transfer across the intact guinea-pig placenta.* J Dev Physiol, 1979. **1**(6): p. 415-26.

56. Dancis, J., V. Jansen, and M. Levitz, *Transfer across perfused human placenta. IV. Effect of protein binding on free fatty acids.* Pediatr Res, 1976. **10**(1): p. 5-10.

57. Dancis, J., et al., *Transfer across perfused human placenta. Effect of chain length on transfer of free fatty acids.* Pediatr Res, 1974. **8**(9): p. 796-9.

58. Rooth, G. and S. Sjostedt, *The placental transfer of gases and fixed acids.* Arch Dis Child, 1962. **37**: p. 366-70.

59. Rattan, S. and J.A. Flaws, *The epigenetic impacts of endocrine disruptors on female reproduction across generations.* Biol Reprod, 2019. **101**(3): p. 635-644.

60. Latchney, S.E., A.M. Fields, and M. Susiarjo, *Linking inter-individual variability to endocrine disruptors: insights for epigenetic inheritance.* Mamm Genome, 2018. **29**(1-2): p. 141-152.

REFERENCES

61. Walker, D.M. and A.C. Gore, *Epigenetic impacts of endocrine disruptors in the brain.* Front Neuroendocrinol, 2017. **44**: p. 1-26.

62. McCabe, C., et al., *Sexually Dimorphic Effects of Early-Life Exposures to Endocrine Disruptors: Sex-Specific Epigenetic Reprogramming as a Potential Mechanism.* Curr Environ Health Rep, 2017. **4**(4): p. 426-438.

63. Skinner, M.K., M. Manikkam, and C. Guerrero-Bosagna, *Epigenetic transgenerational actions of endocrine disruptors.* Reprod Toxicol, 2011. **31**(3): p. 337-43.

64. Doherty, L.F., et al., *In utero exposure to diethylstilbestrol (DES) or bisphenol-A (BPA) increases EZH2 expression in the mammary gland: an epigenetic mechanism linking endocrine disruptors to breast cancer.* Horm Cancer, 2010. **1**(3): p. 146-55.

65. Guerrero-Bosagna, C.M. and M.K. Skinner, *Epigenetic transgenerational effects of endocrine disruptors on male reproduction.* Semin Reprod Med, 2009. **27**(5): p. 403-8.

66. Smith, J. and J. Whitehall, *Sodium valproate and the fetus: a case study and review of the literature.* Neonatal Netw, 2009. **28**(6): p. 363-7.

67. ten Berg, K., et al., *Complex cardiac defect with hypoplastic right ventricle in a fetus with valproate exposure.* Prenat Diagn, 2005. **25**(2): p. 156-8.

68. Berard, A., et al., *SSRI and SNRI use during pregnancy and the risk of persistent pulmonary hypertension of the newborn.* Br J Clin Pharmacol, 2017. **83**(5): p. 1126-1133.

69. *SSRI antidepressants in utero: pulmonary hypertension.* Prescrire Int, 2014. **23**(154): p. 268.

70. *SSRI antidepressants and persistent pulmonary hypertension in newborns.* Prescrire Int, 2008. **17**(96): p. 156.

71. Creasy, R., R. Resnik, and J. Iams, eds. *Maternal -Fetal Medicine: Principles and practice.* 5th ed. 2004, Saunders: Philadelphia.

72. Murphy-Kaulbeck, L., et al., *Single umbilical artery risk factors and pregnancy outcomes.* Obstet Gynecol, 2010. **116**(4): p. 8.

73. Contro, E., et al., *Reference charts for umbilical Doppler pulsatility index in fetuses with isolated two-vessel cord.* Arch Gynecol Obstet, 2019. **299**(4): p. 947-951.

74. Catanzarite, V.A., et al., *Prenatal diagnosis of the two-vessel cord: implications for patient counselling and obstetric management.* Ultrasound Obstet Gynecol, 1995. **5**(2): p. 98-105.

75. Ball, R.H., et al., *The clinical significance of ultransonographically detected subchorionic hemorrhages.* Am J Obstet Gynecol, 1996. **174**(3): p. 996-1002.

76. Kofinas, A.D., et al., *Transabdominal chorionic villus sampling at 9.5-12*

weeks' gestation. Placental vascular resistance and fetal cardiovascular responses. J Reprod Med, 1995. **40**(6): p. 453-7.

77. Milovanov, A.P., et al., *[Uterine pathomorphology in abruptio placentae].* Arkh Patol, 2006. **68**(1): p. 25-7.

78. Balde, M., et al., *[Abruptio placentae].* Geburtshilfe Frauenheilkd, 1990. **50**(3): p. 199-202.

79. Lurie, S., M. Feinstein, and Y. Mamet, *Disseminated intravascular coagulopathy in pregnancy: thorough comprehension of etiology and management reduces obstetricians' stress.* Arch Gynecol Obstet, 2000. **263**(3): p. 126-30.

80. Olah, K.S., H. Gee, and P.G. Needham, *The management of severe disseminated intravascular coagulopathy complicating placental abruption in the second trimester of pregnancy.* Br J Obstet Gynaecol, 1988. **95**(4): p. 419-20.

81. Radakovic, M., M. Toldy, and J. Gajdosova, *[Consumption coagulopathy in pregnancy].* Cesk Gynekol, 1980. **45**(1): p. 36-7.

82. Preston, F.E., et al., *Increased fetal loss in women with heritable thrombophilia.* Lancet, 1996. **348**(9032): p. 913-6.

83. Bick, R.L. and D. Hoppensteadt, *Recurrent miscarriage syndrome and infertility due to blood coagulation protein/platelet defects: a review and update.* Clin Appl Thromb Hemost, 2005. **11**(1): p. 1-13.

84. Gkogkos, P., et al., *Mid-trimester maternal serum AFP levels in predicting adverse pregnancy outcome.* Clin Exp Obstet Gynecol, 2008. **35**(3): p. 208-10.

85. Robinson, L., P. Grau, and B.F. Crandall, *Pregnancy outcomes after increasing maternal serum alpha-fetoprotein levels.* Obstet Gynecol, 1989. **74**(1): p. 17-20.

86. Stirrat, G.M., et al., *Raised maternal serum AFP, oligohydramnios and poor fetal outcome.* Br J Obstet Gynaecol, 1981. **88**(3): p. 231-5.

87. Kjessler, B., et al., *Alpha-fetoprotein (AFP) levels in maternal serum in relation to pregnancy outcome in 7,158 pregnant women prospectively investigated during their 14th-20th week post last menstrual period.* Acta Obstet Gynecol Scand Suppl, 1977. **69**: p. 25-44.

88. Salvig, J.D., et al., *Low PAPP-A in the first trimester is associated with reduced fetal growth rate prior to gestational week 20.* Prenat Diagn, 2010. **30**(6): p. 503-8.

89. Kirkegaard, I., et al., *PAPP-A, free beta-hCG, and early fetal growth identify two pathways leading to preterm delivery.* Prenat Diagn, 2010. **30**(10): p. 956-63.

90. Barrett, S.L., C. Bower, and N.C. Hadlow, *Use of the combined first-trimester screen result and low PAPP-A to predict risk of adverse fetal outcomes.* Prenat Diagn, 2008. **28**(1): p. 28-35.

REFERENCES

91. Spencer, K., et al., *Prediction of pregnancy complications by first-trimester maternal serum PAPP-A and free beta-hCG and with second-trimester uterine artery Doppler.* Prenat Diagn, 2005. **25**(10): p. 949-53.

92. Cuckle, H.S., et al., *Low maternal serum PAPP-A and fetal viability.* Prenat Diagn, 1999. **19**(8): p. 788-90.

93. Chang, S. and T.H. Lee, *Beyond Evidence-Based Medicine.* N Engl J Med, 2018. **379**(21): p. 1983-1985.

94. Ioannidis, J.P.A., *Hijacked evidence-based medicine: stay the course and throw the pirates overboard.* J Clin Epidemiol, 2017. **84**: p. 11-13.

95. Frieden, T.R., *Evidence for Health Decision Making - Beyond Randomized, Controlled Trials.* N Engl J Med, 2017. **377**(5): p. 465-475.

96. Ioannidis, J.P., *Evidence-based medicine has been hijacked: a report to David Sackett.* J Clin Epidemiol, 2016. **73**: p. 82-6.

97. Sackett, D.L., et al., *Evidence based medicine: what it is and what it isn't.* 1996. Clin Orthop Relat Res, 2007. **455**: p. 3-5.

98. Ashcroft, R.E., *Current epistemological problems in evidence based medicine.* J Med Ethics, 2004. **30**(2): p. 131-5.

99. Alfirevic, Z., T. Stampalija, and T. Dowswell, *Fetal and umbilical Doppler ultrasound in high-risk pregnancies.* Cochrane Database Syst Rev, 2017. **6**: p. CD007529.

100. Alfirevic, Z., T. Stampalija, and G.M. Gyte, *Fetal and umbilical Doppler ultrasound in high-risk pregnancies.* Cochrane Database Syst Rev, 2010(1): p. CD007529.

101. Morris, R.K., et al., *Fetal umbilical artery Doppler to predict compromise of fetal/neonatal wellbeing in a high-risk population: systematic review and bivariate meta-analysis.* Ultrasound Obstet Gynecol, 2011. **37**(2): p. 135-42.

102. Morris, R.K., et al., *Systematic review and meta-analysis of the test accuracy of ductus venosus Doppler to predict compromise of fetal/neonatal wellbeing in high risk pregnancies with placental insufficiency.* Eur J Obstet Gynecol Reprod Biol, 2010. **152**(1): p. 3-12.

103. Belfort, M.A., et al., *A Randomized Trial of Intrapartum Fetal ECG ST-Segment Analysis.* N Engl J Med, 2015. **373**(7): p. 632-41.

104. Lalor, J.G., et al., *Biophysical profile for fetal assessment in high risk pregnancies.* Cochrane Database Syst Rev, 2008(1): p. CD000038.

105. Nelson, K.B., et al., *Uncertain value of electronic fetal monitoring in predicting cerebral palsy.* N Engl J Med, 1996. **334**(10): p. 613-8.

106. Leveno, K.J., et al., *A prospective comparison of selective and universal electronic*

fetal monitoring in 34,995 pregnancies. New England Journal of Medicine, 1986. **315**(10): p. 615-9.

107. Kofinas A., B.B., and Kofinas J., *Improved outcomes in ART pregnancies complicated by thrombophilia, treated with low molecular weight heparin in comparison to spontaneously conceived low-risk untreated pregnancies: a case control study.* Obstet Gynecol Int J 2018. **9**(1).

108. Kofinas, A., e.a., *Enoxaparin and Low Dose Aspirin Improve Outcomes in High-Risk Pregnancies Complicated Further by Unexplained Low Maternal Serum Pregnancy-Associated Plasma Protein-A.* EC Gynecology, 2015. **1**(3): p. 8.

109. Kofinas, A., *Standard-of-Care in Obstetrics: An Advantage or A Hindrance?* EC Gynecology, 2015. **2**(3): p. 4.

110. Cusimano, M.C., et al., *The maternal health clinic: an initiative for cardiovascular risk identification in women with pregnancy-related complications.* Am J Obstet Gynecol, 2014. **210**(5): p. 438 e1-9.

111. Smith, G.N., J. Pudwell, and M. Roddy, *The Maternal Health Clinic: a new window of opportunity for early heart disease risk screening and intervention for women with pregnancy complications.* J Obstet Gynaecol Can, 2013. **35**(9): p. 831-839.

112. Pell, J.P., G.C. Smith, and D. Walsh, *Pregnancy complications and subsequent maternal cerebrovascular events: a retrospective cohort study of 119,668 births.* Am J Epidemiol, 2004. **159**(4): p. 336-42.

113. Smith, G.C., J.P. Pell, and D. Walsh, *Pregnancy complications and maternal risk of ischaemic heart disease: a retrospective cohort study of 129,290 births.* Lancet, 2001. **357**(9273): p. 2002-6.

114. Zhang, Y., *Cardiovascular diseases in American women.* Nutr Metab Cardiovasc Dis, 2010. **20**(6): p. 386-93.

115. Qublan, H.S., et al., *Acquired and inherited thrombophilia: implication in recurrent IVF and embryo transfer failure.* Hum Reprod, 2006. **21**(10): p. 2694-8.

116. Ariel, I., et al., *Placental pathology in fetal thrombophilia.* Hum Pathol, 2004. **35**(6): p. 729-33.

117. Bloomenthal, D., et al., *The effect of factor V Leiden carriage on maternal and fetal health.* Cmaj, 2002. **167**(1): p. 48-54.

118. Khong, T.Y. and W.M. Hague, *Biparental contribution to fetal thrombophilia in discordant twin intrauterine growth restriction.* Am J Obstet Gynecol, 2001. **185**(1): p. 244-5.

119. Leistra-Leistra, M.J., et al., *Fetal thrombotic vasculopathy in the placenta: a thrombophilic connection between pregnancy complications and neonatal thrombosis?* Placenta, 2004. **25 Suppl A**: p. S102-5.

REFERENCES

120. Vefring, H., et al., *Maternal and fetal variants of genetic thrombophilias and the risk of preeclampsia.* Epidemiology, 2004. **15**(3): p. 317-22.

121. Barcellona, D., et al., *Allele 4G of gene PAI-1 associated with prothrombin mutation G20210A increases the risk for venous thrombosis.* Thromb Haemost, 2003. **90**(6): p. 1061-4.

122. Mello, G., et al., *Low-molecular-weight heparin lowers the recurrence rate of preeclampsia and restores the physiological vascular changes in angiotensin-converting enzyme DD women.* Hypertension, 2005. **45**(1): p. 86-91.

123. Aracic, N., et al., *The Impact of Inherited Thrombophilia Types and Low Molecular Weight Heparin Treatment on Pregnancy Complications in Women with Previous Adverse Outcome.* Yonsei Med J, 2016. **57**(5): p. 1230-5.

124. Segui, R., et al., *PAI-1 promoter 4G/5G genotype as an additional risk factor for venous thrombosis in subjects with genetic thrombophilic defects.* Br J Haematol, 2000. **111**(1): p. 122-8.

125. Gris, J.C., et al., *Low-molecular-weight heparin versus low-dose aspirin in women with one fetal loss and a constitutional thrombophilic disorder.* Blood, 2004. **103**(10): p. 3695-9.

126. Paidas, M.J., et al., *Protein Z, protein S levels are lower in patients with thrombophilia and subsequent pregnancy complications.* J Thromb Haemost, 2005. **3**(3): p. 497-501.

127. Bretelle, F., et al., *Protein Z in patients with pregnancy complications.* Am J Obstet Gynecol, 2005. **193**(5): p. 1698-702.

128. Bartholomew, R.A., *Pathology of the placenta: with special reference to infarcts and their relation to toxaemia of pregnancy.* Journal of the American Medical Association, 1938. **111**: p. 2276-2280.

129. Redline, R.W., *Clinical and pathological umbilical cord abnormalities in fetal thrombotic vasculopathy.* Hum Pathol, 2004. **35**(12): p. 1494-8.

130. P., G., *Abnormalities of placental vascularity in relation to intrauterine deprivation and retardation of fetal growth: significance of avascular villi.* New York State J Med., 1961. **61**: p. 6.

131. McDermott, M. and J.E. Gillan, *Chronic reduction in fetal blood flow is associated with placental infarction.* Placenta, 1995. **16**(2): p. 165-70.

132. Shastri, M.D., et al., *Opposing effects of low molecular weight heparins on the release of inflammatory cytokines from peripheral blood mononuclear cells of asthmatics.* PLoS One, 2015. **10**(3): p. e0118798.

133. Hochart, H., et al., *Low-molecular weight and unfractionated heparins induce a downregulation of inflammation: decreased levels of proinflammatory cytokines and nuclear*

factor-kappaB in LPS-stimulated human monocytes. Br J Haematol, 2006. **133**(1): p. 62-67.

134. Sobel, M.L., J. Kingdom, and S. Drewlo, *Angiogenic response of placental villi to heparin.* Obstet Gynecol, 2011. **117**(6): p. 1375-83.

135. Nagy, S., et al., *Clinical significance of subchorionic and retroplacental hematomas detected in the first trimester of pregnancy.* Obstet Gynecol, 2003. **102**(1): p. 94-100.

136. Maso, G., et al., *First-trimester intrauterine hematoma and outcome of pregnancy.* Obstet Gynecol, 2005. **105**(2): p. 339-44.

137. Johns, J., J. Hyett, and E. Jauniaux, *Obstetric outcome after threatened miscarriage with and without a hematoma on ultrasound.* Obstet Gynecol, 2003. **102**(3): p. 483-7.

138. Gianpaolo M., e.a., *First-trimester intrauterine hematoma and outcome of pregnancy.* Obstet Gynecol, 2005. **105**(2): p. 6.

139. Jivraj, S., et al., *Genetic thrombophilic mutations among couples with recurrent miscarriage.* Hum Reprod, 2006. **21**(5): p. 1161-5.

140. Hohlagschwandtner, M., et al., *Combined thrombophilic polymorphisms in women with idiopathic recurrent miscarriage.* Fertil Steril, 2003. **79**(5): p. 1141-8.

141. Douketis J.D., K.K., and Crowther M.A., *Anticoagulant effect at the time of epidural catheter removal in patients receiving twice-daily or once-daily low-molecular-weight heparin and continuous epidural analgesia after orthopedic surgery.* Thromb Haemost, 2002. **88**: p. 4.

142. Casele, H.L., et al., *Changes in the pharmacokinetics of the low-molecular-weight heparin enoxaparin sodium during pregnancy.* Am J Obstet Gynecol, 1999. **181**(5 Pt 1): p. 1113-7.

143. Fox, N.S., et al., *Anti-factor Xa plasma levels in pregnant women receiving low molecular weight heparin thromboprophylaxis.* Obstet Gynecol, 2008. **112**(4): p. 884-9.

144. Hamilton, B.E., et al., *Annual summary of vital statistics: 2010-2011.* Pediatrics, 2013. **131**(3): p. 548-58.

145. Kim, Y.M., et al., *Failure of physiologic transformation of the spiral arteries in the placental bed in preterm premature rupture of membranes.* Am J Obstet Gynecol, 2002. **187**(5): p. 1137-42.

146. Kim, Y.M., et al., *Failure of physiologic transformation of the spiral arteries in patients with preterm labor and intact membranes.* Am J Obstet Gynecol, 2003. **189**(4): p. 1063-9.

147. McMaster-Fay, R.A., *Failure of physiologic transformation of the spiral arteries of the uteroplacental circulation in patients with preterm labor and intact membranes.* Am J Obstet Gynecol, 2004. **191**(5): p. 1837-8; author reply 1838-9.

REFERENCES

148. Mercer, B.M., *Preterm premature rupture of the membranes: diagnosis and management.* Clin Perinatol, 2004. **31**(4): p. 765-82, vi.

149. Phibbs, C.S. and S.K. Schmitt, *Estimates of the cost and length of stay changes that can be attributed to one-week increases in gestational age for premature infants.* Early Hum Dev, 2006. **82**(2): p. 85-95.

150. Little, W.J., *On the influence of abnormal parturition, difficult labours, premature birth, and asphyxia neonatorum, on the mental and physical condition of the child, especially in relation to deformities.* Trans Obstet Soc (London), 1862. **3**(293): p. 16.

151. Behrman, R.E., et al., *Distribution of the circulation in the normal and asphyxiated fetal primate.* Am J Obstet Gynecol, 1970. **108**(6): p. 956-69.

152. Wladimiroff, J.W., et al., *Cerebral and umbilical arterial blood flow velocity waveforms in normal and growth-retarded pregnancies.* Obstet Gynecol, 1987. **69**(5): p. 705-9.

153. Bonnin, A., et al., *A transient placental source of serotonin for the fetal forebrain.* Nature, 2011. **472**(7343): p. 347-50.

154. McKay, R., *Developmental biology: Remarkable role for the placenta.* Nature, 2011. **472**(7343): p. 298-9.

155. St-Pierre, J., et al., *Effects of prenatal maternal stress on serotonin and fetal development.* Placenta, 2016. **40 Suppl 1**: p S66-S71.

156. Musumeci, G., et al., *Serotonin (5HT) expression in rat pups treated with high-tryptophan diet during fetal and early postnatal development.* Acta Histochem, 2014. **116**(2): p. 335-43.

157. Houlihan, J., et al., *https://www.ewg.org/research/body-burden-pollution-newborns.* Environmental Working Group, 2005.

158. Alfirevic, Z., Devane D., Gyte GML., *Continuous cardiotocography (CTG) as a form of electronic fetal monitoring (EFM) for fetal assessment during labour.* Cochrane Database of Systematic Reviews, 2008(4).

159. Graham, E.M., et al., *Intrapartum electronic fetal heart rate monitoring and the prevention of perinatal brain injury.* Obstet Gynecol, 2006. **108**(3 Pt 1): p. 656-66.

160. Greene, M.F., *Obstetricians still await a deus ex machina.* N Engl J Med, 2006. **355**(21): p. 2247-8.

161. Kofinas, A.D., et al., *Functional asymmetry of the human myometrium documented by color and pulsed-wave Doppler ultrasonographic evaluation of uterine arcuate arteries during Braxton Hicks contractions.* Am J Obstet Gynecol, 1993. **168**(1 Pt 1): p. 184-8.

162. Kofinas, A.D., et al., *Effect of placental laterality on uterine artery resistance and development of preeclampsia and intrauterine growth retardation.* Am J Obstet Gynecol,

1989. **161**(6 Pt 1): p. 1536-9.

163. Kofinas, A.D., et al., *Interrelationship and clinical significance of increased resistance in the uterine arteries in patients with hypertension or preeclampsia or both.* Am J Obstet Gynecol, 1992. **166**(2): p. 601-6.

164. Kofinas, A.D., et al., *The effect of placental location on uterine artery flow velocity waveforms.* Am J Obstet Gynecol, 1988. **159**(6): p. 1504-8.

165. Guaschino, S., et al., *Assessment of peri-neonatal mortality and morbidity risk in twin pregnancy.* Clin Exp Obstet Gynecol, 1986. **13**(1-2): p. 18-25.

About the Author

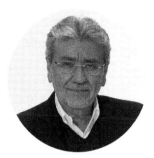

ALEXANDER KOFINAS, MD, has won many awards, including New York magazine Best Doctor (eight times), Patient Choice and Most Compassionate Doctor, and has published dozens of scientific papers. A textbook co-author, he's also an academic reviewer for the American Journal of Obstetrics & Gynecology, Journal of Perinatology, Journal of Ultrasound in Medicine, Journal of Maternal-Fetal & Neonatal Medicine, Journal of Pregnancy, Obstetrics & Gynecology, Hypertension in Pregnancy, and the authoritative medical journal Placenta. He studied at Athens University, Greece; Good Samaritan Hospital, Cincinnati, OH; Brooklyn and Caledonian Hospitals, NY; and Bowman Gray School of Medicine, Wake Forest U, NC. He's been Director of Maternal-Fetal Medicine and Associate Director, Obstetrics/Gynecology Residency Program, at York Hospital, PA, and Chief, Maternal-Fetal Medicine, at Brooklyn Hospital Center, NY. Since 2000, he's led Kofinas Perinatal PC's clinics in Manhattan, Brooklyn and Garden City, NY. Since 2003, he's been Associate Professor of Clinical Obstetrics & Gynecology, Weill Cornell Medicine, Cornell University, NY. He's also been Assistant Professor of Clinical Obstetrics & Gynecology, NYU, and taught at U Penn and Wake Forest U, NC. Certified by the American Board of Obstetrics & Gynecology (Div of Maternal-Fetal Medicine), he's licensed in NY, PA, NC and MD and is a member of the American Society for Reproductive Medicine, American Society for Reproductive Immunology, American College of Angiology, International Society of Ultrasound in Obstetrics & Gynecology, International Society of Perinatal Obstetricians, Society for Maternal-Fetal Medicine, American Institute of Ultrasound in Medicine, American Medical Association, American College of Obstetricians & Gynecologists, Athens Medical Association and International Federation of Placenta Associations.

Printed in Poland
by Amazon Fulfillment
Poland Sp. z o.o., Wrocław